A Natural Approach

DIABETES and HYPOGLYCEMIA

Macrobiotic Health Education Series

D1563010

MACROBIOTIC HEALTH EDUCATION SERIES

A Natural Approach

Diabetes
and
Hypoglycemia

by Michio Kushi

edited by John David Mann

foreword by Marc Van Cauwenberghe, M. D.

Japan Publications, Inc.

Tokyo • New York

Note to the reader: Those with health problems are advised to seek the guidance
of a qualified medical, or psychological professional in addition to qualified
macrobiotic counselor before implementing any of the dietary and other approaches presented in this book. It is essential that any reader who has any
reason to suspect serious illness in themselves or their family members seek
appropriate medical, nutritional, or psychological advice promptly. Neither this
or any other health related book should be used as a substitute for qualified
care or treatment.

Published by JAPAN PUBLICATIONS, INC., Tokyo and New York

Distributors:
UNITED STATES: *Kodansha International/USA, Ltd., through Harper & Row,
Publishers, Inc., 10 East 53rd Street, New York, New York 10022.* SOUTH AMERICA:
Harper & Row, Publishers, Inc., International Department. CANADA: *Fitzhenry
& Whiteside Ltd., 195 Allstate Parkway, Markham, Ontario, L3R 4T8.* MEXICO
AND CENTRAL AMERICA: *HARLA S. A. de C. V., Apartado 30–546, Mexico 4,
D. F.* BRITISH ISLES: *International Book Distributors Ltd., 66 Wood Lane End,
Hemel Hempstead, Herts HP2 4RG.* EUROPEAN CONTINENT: *Fleetbooks, S. A.,
c/o Feffer and Simons (Nederland) B. V., Rijnkade 170, 1382 GT Weesp, The
Netherlands.* AUSTRALIA AND NEW ZEALAND: *Bookwise International, 1 Jeanes
Street, Beverley, South Australia 5007.* THE FAR EAST AND JAPAN: *Japan Publi-
cations Trading Co., Ltd., 1–2–1, Sarugaku-cho, Chiyoda-ku, Tokyo 101.*

First edition: April 1985

LCCC No. 84–081356
ISBN 0–87040–615–9

Printed in U.S.A.

Foreword

Fourteen years have passed since I started practicing the macrobiotic way of living. I am now convinced that this very practical way contains the solution, and probably the only solution, for present day mankind's problem—physical, mental, social, and spiritual.

I graduated as an M.D. in 1969, together with 88 colleagues. Since that time several of these colleague physicians have developed chronic illnesses such as diabetes and chronic allergies, and one has already died of rectal cancer. When I meet them now, several look many years older than their real age.

After becoming macrobiotic, I started to gain hundreds of new friends, also living macrobiotically. Among all friends who are correctly practicing the macrobiotic way of eating, and who have continued their study of macrobiotics, I know of no one who has developed diabetes, allergies, or cancer in the past 10 years. Many of them look much younger than their real age, and most of them actually look better than 10 years ago.

Modern medicine knows very well that diabetes has everything to do with modern way of eating. A diabetologist recently stated that "Diabetes patients are victims of a genetic apparatus which is not yet adapted to a superfluous way of living; therefore their metabolism cannot handle excess." In other words, if they and their immediate ancestors would have lived in a less modern environment, they would never have developed diabetes. Similarly wild animals do not seem to develop diabetes often, while it is not rare among domesticated animals.

George Ohsawa, the man who reinterpreted macrobiotics, called the macrobiotic way of life *vivere parvo*: "live with little." Fifteen years ago I detested this statement, because I interpreted this as "live in poverty," and I did not like poverty. But what Mr. Ohsawa meant was: try not to live from luxuries which are unnatural and unnecessary for life. We can enjoy our lives and be happy by eating simple foods such as brown rice, dark bread, unpeeled vegetables, sea vegetables or wild vegetables. In this sense macrobiotics is not another diet for the diabetic, but a return to the original way of eating of all mankind.

In my experience, people suffering from diabetes who discover and practice macrobiotics become much happier and can live a healthy life.

If they are taking insulin, they often feel the need to reduce their dosage. Usually they can eventually reduce it 70% to 100%. But most of all they are happy because they practice a macrobiotic way of eating which they feel they can easily maintain for the rest of their lives.

MARC VAN CAUWENBERGHE, M.D.

Brookline, Massachusetts
November, 1984

Introduction ▬▬▬▬▬▬▬▬▬

Our purpose in presenting the *Macrobiotic Health Education Series* is two-fold. The primary concern, of course, has been to present the reader with the practical application of macrobiotic principles, through daily eating and lifestyle, to a broad range of specific health problems. In contrast to the modern trend towards specialization, the macrobiotic approach to health aims at nourishing and restoring the whole person to a naturally healthy, happy condition on all levels, including physical, emotional, mental and spiritual well-being. Because of this holistic scope, the practice of macrobiotics is naturally applicable to the widest range of different health problems. Macrobiotics, indeed, can be adapted to help alleviate virtually any aspect of human suffering, provided that appropriate modifications for each individual illness or circumstance are introduced with the proper understanding.

At the same time, the ancient unifying principle of yin and yang can be applied as a practical approach to studying and clarifying the various scientific riddles in a problem such as *diabetes* and *hypoglycemia,* and offers a clear understanding of the origin, cause and mechanism of each problem under study.

On a broader level, each particular problem addressed in the *Health Education Series* also illustrates larger issues underlying our modern civilization's orientation, way of thinking and approach to life. By examining such philosophical questions, the *Health Education Series* is also presenting the larger goal of macrobiotics, which is to establish health at the individual, family and community levels as a first step towards solving larger social and national problems and, eventually, helping to create a firm foundation for health, happiness and peace on a global scale.

The problem of diabetes and hypoglycemia presents three interesting philosophical issues. First, the entire problem of blood glucose disorders is directly related to our modern diet and its departure from the traditional staples of whole cereal grains, fresh local vegetables and other complex carbohydrate foods. As our diet has steadily lost its center and shifted towards greater and greater extremes, the problems of diabetes and hypoglycemia have escalated proportionately. This raises a question of lifestyle and values, namely those of more traditional moderation versus the more

8

modern tendency towards extremes in general.

Second, our inability to stem the tide of diabetes over the past half-century points to the limitation of purely symptomatic approaches to human problems, and to the need for a broader and more fundamental understanding.

Finally, nutritional approaches to diabetes have in recent years developed to the point where they closely parallel macrobiotic dietary guidelines in many ways. As described in Chapter Five, for example, the official nutritional guidelines currently offered by the American Diabetes Association represent a radical departure from the earlier diets high in fat, protein and animal foods, and towards more complex carbohydrate foods and even vegetarianism or semi-vegetarianism. In other words, we have already entered an era where science will more easily adapt macrobiotic principles and practices in its efforts to find solutions to our multiple ills.

The few anecdotal case histories presented in this volume represent only a sampling of the many such cases of improvement and recovery through macrobiotics we have witnessed over the past thirty years since macrobiotics has been introduced and developed in the Western world. During this time, the development of the macrobiotic movement has grown to encompass a broad range of educational activities, including a network of several hundred educational centers throughout the United States, Canada, western Europe, South America and the Far East, as well as in parts of eastern Europe, Africa, Australia and other countries. In the U.S. alone, over 15,000 natural foods, health foods and other stores now carry macrobiotic staple food supplies and literature on the macrobiotic approach to health. The basic tenets of the macrobiotic health approach have also begun to appear in major health agencies' research reports, such as the 1977 U.S. Senate report *Dietary Goals for the United States* and the 1982 National Research Council's report on *Diet, Nutrition and Cancer*. More recently, many medical doctors and scientific agencies have begun to work in collaboration with macrobiotic organizations such as the East West Foundation on research projects to document scientifically the efficacy of the mactobiotic approach in relieving illness.

We would like to thank all of the people who have contributed to these first volumes of the *Health Education Series*. We thank Iwao Yoshizaki, President of Japan Publications, Inc., and Yoshiro Fujiwara, the Japan Publications representative for America, for their guidance and advice, together with our macrobiotic associate Edward Esko. We also thank Phillip Janetta in Tokyo for editing the final text, and Peter and Bonnie Harris for providing the illustrations. Our gratitude also goes to Marc Van Cauwenberghe, M.D., for contributing the Foreword, and to all of our friends who wrote case histories. We also thank Aveline Kushi, Rosalind

Rhodes, Olivia Oredson and Wendy Esko for their efforts in developing the companion volume in the *Macrobiotic Food and Cooking Series, Cooking for Diabetes and Hypoglycemia.*

Everything changes, eventually, into its opposite; and just as the darkest night contains the seeds of a newly unfolding dawn, the modern trend towards degeneration, burgeoning social confusion and geo-political dangers carries within it the hopes for a new world of peace and health. If a simple, natural model for solving the problems of diabetes and hypoglycemia may be followed as one example, this turning point may be soon at hand.

MICHIO KUSHI
JOHN DAVID MANN

Brookline, Massachusetts
November, 1984

Contents

1. Diet, Nutrition and the Sugar Disorders━━━

At the beginning of this century diabetes was a rare, virtually untreatable disease; its companion disorder, hypoglycemia, had not yet even been identified. Over the past eighty years, these two metabolic problems have burst upon the populations of modernized societies with all the force of an epidemic. In the thirty-seven years from 1936 to 1973, for example, diabetes rose from our twelfth leading cause of death to rank seventh, where it still stands today. At the onset of World War II about one million Americans had diabetes. Today there are at least eleven times, and possibly as many as twenty times that number. This figure is increasing at an annual rate of 6 percent and costs a staggering $15.7 billion each year.[1]

Together with cancer, cardiovascular illness and other problems, diabetes is part of a widespread degenerative trend pervading modern life. Like diabetes, most of such chronic illnesses have escalated from relative obscurity to a frightening prominence within the 20th century. One out of every five Americans born during 1984 is expected to have diabetes; two out of every five living today will die from heart or artery disease, and every third person living today is expected to have cancer at some time in their lives. Adding together the statistics for these and other similar health problems suggests that virtually nobody is untouched by this biological Noah's flood. If these trends are not reversed soon, the very existence of the modern human population may well be threatened within another thirty to forty years.

In the past several years, this alarming trend has prompted a mood of sober, broad-ranging self-reflection throughout society at large, in the public media, and particularly within the medical and research communities. The dramatic increase of diabetes, in particular, has resulted over the last two decades in one of the most extensive research campaigns in medical history. Since the development of insulin injection therapy in the 1920's, great strides have been made in describing what is actually happening in the course of the disease. Research has led to improved longer-acting insulins, to oral antidiabetic drugs in the 1950's, and to substantial improvement in nutritional understanding in the 1970's.

Yet there is scarcely any better understanding now of why diabetes develops than there was eighty years ago. And despite the widely heralded new era brought about by insulin therapy and other developments, the incidence and mortality rates from this illness continue to climb. At the rate of one death every two minutes, diabetes claims over 340,000 lives annually—just over 1/2 the death rate of cancer—and over twice that many new cases are discovered each year. Since you began reading this chapter, two new cases of diabetes developed, and one person died from its effects.

Regarding the mysterious companion problem of hypoglycemia, the situation is far more obscure but hardly less devastating. There is still some controversy within scientific and medical circles as to whether the disorder even exists to any large degree, and there is considerable dispute as to the correct methods and guidelines for diagnosis. Yet, according to the Hypoglycemia Foundation, conservative estimates place the current incidence at between 10 and 25 percent of the population,[2] and one U. S. Government survey has suggested that hypoglycemia may afflict nearly one half the population.[3] Though there is virtually no direct mortality rate, the number of deaths due to disorders that are commonly linked with hypoglycemia, such as alcoholism, suicide and violent crime, suggests that the "darker side" of blood glucose imbalance may exact as fierce (or fiercer) a toll on modern health and happiness as its more clearly identified sister, diabetes.

Within the growing circle of practicing nutritionists and nutritionally aware physicians, substantial progress has been made in recognizing and diagnosing hypoglycemia. But again, no satisfactory explanation has been advanced as to exactly why the problem exists, or precisely how it develops. Such treatment as there is often fails to adequately solve the problem. Like insulin or drug therapy for diabetes, treatment for hypoglycemia, through nutrition, nutritional supplementation or hormone therapy, sometimes alleviates symptoms temporarily, but offers no lasting cure.

What compounds the sheer magnitude of these health problems, therefore, is the increasingly apparent fact that conventional medical research and treatments have not been able to keep pace with the growing rate of their appearance. In general, the direction of medical research and treatment has been microscopic, often to the exclusion of the macroscopic. This is to say, their efforts tend to focus on the minute biochemical or genetic details of the disease process, and lack a clear view of the larger context within which that process is led to occur.

This relative failure on the part of modern science to cope effectively with the problems of carbohydrate metabolic disorders stems from fundamental limitations of the present scientific approach, which is lacking in a clear understanding of human life, health and sickness. The term "peace," for example, is currently used to describe the absence of openly armed hostilities; actually, such temporary periods are usually far from peaceful, and are fraught with the uneasy tensions that inevitably erupt again into war. In the same way, true health is far more than the temporary absence of clearly symptomatic disease—what is often thought of as "health" today all too easily erupts suddenly and unexpectedly into heart attack, stroke, cancer or diabetes.

To stem the tide of chronic, debilitating illnesses, the observation and treatment of individual symptoms needs to be complemented by a more comprehensive approach to health and life itself. This broader approach lay at the core of all older, more traditional healing disciplines prior to the past several hundred years, including ancient Chinese and Indian medicine, the medicine of Hippocrates (the Father of Western Medicine), and others. This wider view is represented in the modern age by the rediscovery, updating and further development of such approaches going under the name "macrobiotics." From the Greek "makro" (large) and "bios" (life), the term *macrobiotics* has been used throughout the ages to describe a natural approach to diet and daily living, aimed at achieving longevity and harmony within the self and with the larger context of the natural world. It is with this larger view of life that our understanding of diabetes and hypoglycemia begins.

The Source of Life

While the modern view of health focuses on the body and its intricate biochemical processes, the macrobiotic approach takes the opposite perspective, beginning with the broadest possible view of the natural environment within which our life is created and sustained. From this larger perspective, we can clearly see that the sun, sky and soil around us are as essential to human life as our own hearts, brains and bloodstreams. If deprived of any of these natural functions, we would cease to exist. In this sense, we can consider the natural surroundings as our "outer body" and our physiological selves as our "inner body."

Health, then, can be described as the active, harmonious dialogue between both spheres of life. The attempt to understand sickness only through painstaking observations of the body's workings inevitably falls short of its goals; for the bodily symptoms of disease are only the results of sickness, not the origin. The root causes of sickness, like those of health, lie ultimately in how we are deriving our nourishment from this larger body.

We are in constant exchange with our environment, absorbing nourishment on every level from solid food, liquids and inhaled gasses to heat, light, and the full range of vibrations and waves filling our atmosphere. At the same time, we are perpetually giving our nourishments back out to our surroundings, in the form of solid and liquid waste, exhaled carbon dioxide (CO_2), caloric heat and the vibrations of our expression and behavior.

There is a grand symmetry in this process, reflecting the natural order of the universe in which seemingly opposed forces actually support one another through co-operative exchange. For example, we require oxygen for our cells' activities; and from those activities we generate CO_2, which to us is a poison. To the plant world, though, that same CO_2 is a necessity, and as vegetation thrives on that gas it generates its own "poison"—the oxygen so vital to our existence. This harmonious exchange between animal and vegetable kingdoms, further, is reflected in the larger exchange between biological life as a whole and the realm of the natural elements.

The substances that create and nourish us are derived primarily from the sun's energy, which combines with elements in our natural environment to give us form—in essence, we are nothing but phantoms, transformations of sun, sky, rain and soil. But we cannot absorb these environmental forces directly, and for this we must rely on the plant world. Plants have the unique capacity to tie up solar energy into physical packages that animals can then use. This is another illustration of the beautifully co-operative exchange between vegetable and animal kingdoms. Whether directly or by consuming other plant-eating creatures, all animal life depends on vegetal life. In this sense, plants are our parents, and the elements our grandparents.

Yin and Yang

The contrasting but cooperative behavior of the plant and animal kingdoms extends beyond the exchange of gasses. Plants, for example, grow their roots out into the soil, while we carry our "roots" internally in the intestine where our nutrients are absorbed. While a plant's respiratory system—its leaves—expands up and outward, our lungs are compacted and internal. Plants are stationary while we are active and mobile. Thus, vegetal and animal life are dominated by opposing, balancing forces, which we can call *yin* and *yang*. Yin, representing a more quiet, passive and centrifugally expanding tendency, is more characteristic of plants, while yang, a more active, contracting and centripetal tendency, describes animals. The cycle of gasses and nourishment between the two is an expression of the natural attraction between opposites, similar to the polar relationship between the sexes, the positive and negative electrical poles, or the interaction of light and shade in a great painting.

These are all examples of yin and yang. All phenomena in the universe, in fact, are perpetually moving through cycles of attraction and change, guided by the mutually opposing yet harmonizing tendencies of yin and yang. Figure 2 illustrates some common examples of yin and yang, and will serve to introduce you to this simple yet profoundly comprehensive way of looking at the world.[4]

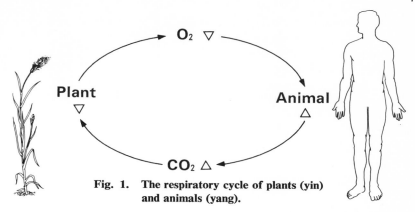

Fig. 1.   The respiratory cycle of plants (yin) and animals (yang).

Like the turning of the tides and seasons, all events in nature strive for harmony by balancing their relative degrees of yin and yang qualities. In terms of human health, this suggests that our diet should on the whole rely as little as possible on animal foods, and more on vegetable foods. Further, we unconsciously strive to balance yin and yang qualities within our foods. A quick glance at Figure 3 reveals that consuming foods that are more extremely yang naturally leads to a desire for more yin foods, resulting in common pairings such as steak and ice cream, eggs and orange juice or cheese and wine. However, a diet based on such extremes exacts its toll on our health. Eating foods with a more moderate, mild tendency is easier to balance and places less wear and tear on the body, and is the central principle of macrobiotic eating. If we eat largely vegetable foods, and balance their different qualities properly, we tend to achieve more of a natural harmony between both our inner and outer selves, or our physiology and our environment. We will explore this idea in more detail later on; for now, we can direct our attention to the food at the center of the chart, the most centrally balanced food, whole cereal grains.

The Staff of Life

Over the centuries, humanity has evolved a way of eating that very efficiently maintains this balance. Throughout the world, differences in climate, terrain and the availability of certain foods, as well as cultural and ethnic customs, have produced a rich diversity of local cuisine. Yet, underlying these apparent differences, there is a surprisingly uniform pattern wherever the traditional, indigenous way of eating prevails.[5]

In nearly every region and time in history, the role of whole grains as a staple food has been the central pillar of this universal dietary practice. As well as being an easily stored and nutritionally balanced food staple, grain crops adapt to virtually any growing climate or season, and make very efficient use of arable land. Also widely regarded as a potent healing force, whole grains formed the core of the medical dietary therapies of physicians such as Hippocrates in Greece and Ch'i Po (the "Yellow Emperor") in China.

Fig. 2. Examples of yin and yang phenomena.

General	YIN ▽ * Centrifugal force	YANG △ * Centripetal force
Tendency	Expansion	Contraction
Function	Diffusion	Fusion
	Dispersion	Assimilation
	Separation	Gathering
	Decomposition	Organization
Movement	More inactive and slower	More active and faster
Vibration	Shorter wave and high frequency	Longer wave and low frequency
Direction	Ascent and vertical	Descent and horizontal
Position	More outward and peripheral	More inward and central
Weight	Lighter	Heavier
Temperature	Colder	Hotter
Light	Darker	Brighter
Humidity	More wet	More dry
Density	Thinner	Thicker
Size	Longer	Smaller
Shape	More expansive and fragile	More contractive and harder
Form	Longer	Shorter
Texture	Softer	Harder
Atomic particle	Electron	Proton
Elements	N, O, K, P, Ca, etc.	H, C, Na, As, Mg, etc.
Environment	Vibration . . . Air . . . Water . . . Earth	
Climatic effects	Tropical climate	Colder climate
Biological	More vegetable quality	More animal quality
Sex	Female	Male
Organ structure	More hollow and expansive	More compacted and condensed
Nerves	More peripheral, ortho-sympathetic	More central, para-sympathetic
Attitude	More gentle, negative	More active, positive
Work	More psychological and mental	More physical and social
Dimension	Space	Time

* For convenience, the symbols ▽ for Yin, and △ for Yang are used.
Source: The Book of Macrobiotics, Tokyo; Japan Publications, 1977.

Fig. 3. Examples of foods as generally classified by yin and yang.

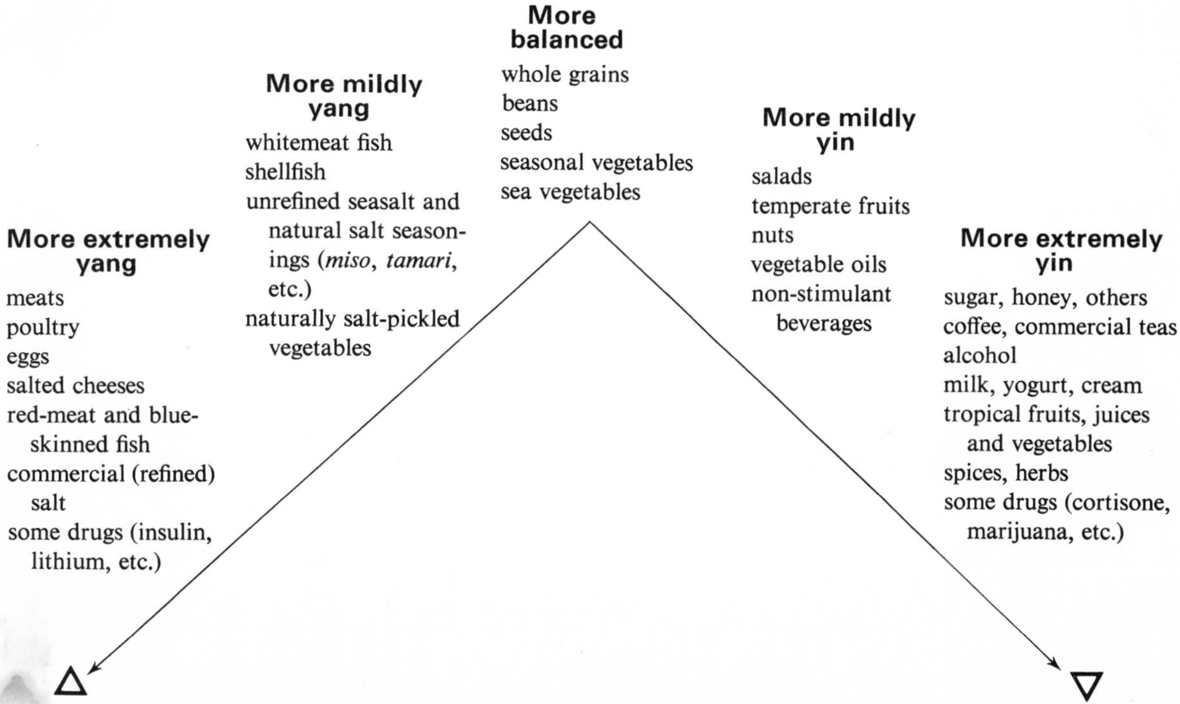

More extremely yang

meats
poultry
eggs
salted cheeses
red-meat and blue-skinned fish
commercial (refined) salt
some drugs (insulin, lithium, etc.)

More mildly yang

whitemeat fish
shellfish
unrefined seasalt and natural salt season-ings (*miso, tamari,* etc.)
naturally salt-pickled vegetables

More balanced

whole grains
beans
seeds
seasonal vegetables
sea vegetables

More mildly yin

salads
temperate fruits
nuts
vegetable oils
non-stimulant beverages

More extremely yin

sugar, honey, others
coffee, commercial teas
alcohol
milk, yogurt, cream
tropical fruits, juices and vegetables
spices, herbs
some drugs (cortisone, marijuana, etc.)

To the ecologically attuned sensibilities of traditional peoples, whole grains represented far more than a source of dietary energy—grains came to assume a central role in practically every aspect of daily life, including diet, agriculture, medicine, language, culture and economy. For example, rice and millet were principal foods in the Orient; wheat, oats and rye in Europe; buckwheat (*kasha*) in Russia and central Asia; sorghum in Africa; barley in the middle East; and corn in the Americas. In fact, the English word for food is *meal* or ground grain, and in Japan the term for a meal is *gohan*, meaning "cooked rice."

The special relationship of whole cereals and human life also has an evolutionary basis. Over the course of development of biological life on the Earth, each animal species has emerged together with the plant forms upon which it primarily depends. For example, the larger dinosaurs could only co-exist with the gigantic, lush foliage of their era, while the smaller, more dense forms of modern vegetable plants, nuts, seeds and fruits gave rise to families of mammals, squirrels, birds and apes. The most recent arrivals, and the most complex, have been the cereals and the human family. Thus, while our highly evolved systems are capable of consuming virtually any form of life as food, grains have naturally continued to serve as our primary link with the sun, soil, and our own human biological heritage.[6]

Seen in nutritional terms, whole grains and other foods more to the center of the spectrum of yin and yang are higher in complex carbohydrate. Many of the more extremely yin foods are higher in simple carbohydrates ("simple sugars"), and the more extremely yang foods contain virtually no carbohydrate at all, but more fat and protein. When we examine the traditional dietary pattern, we discover that it reflects a more centrally balanced order in these terms as well.

1. *Carbohydrates:* The bulk of food energy has universally been supplied by the complex carbohydrates or starch group, supplemented by smaller proportions of foods higher in protein, fat and simple sugars. Whole, unrefined cereal grains, such as whole wheat, whole (brown) rice, oats and barley, have been the primary source of carbohydrate, with a variety of fresh, seasonal vegetables (usually cooked) as the second major source.

2. *Protein*: Traditionally comprising a much smaller proportion of the diet, protein has been supplied in the form of whole grains, dried beans, seeds and nuts, which also contain some vegetable fats (oils) as well as some amount of polysaccharide.

3. *Fat*: A small amount of fat is necessary in the human diet for normal

metabolism, and this has been supplied, when climate conditions permit, in more unsaturated form as oil contained in whole grains, beans, seeds, nuts and various vegetables. In colder climates, somewhat more fats or oils are often needed; however saturated or animal fats have been relied on far less than in present modern eating, and fats as a whole have comprised a far smaller portion of the traditional diet than in common present-day practice.

4. *Vitamins and Minerals*: Vitamins and minerals have been supplied in refined or supplement form only in this century, with the increased refining of foods and more extreme food preferences. The traditional diet, including a wider variety of fresh, unprocessed or naturally prepared foods, has generally provided all the essential micro-nutrients necessary for normal human health.

5. *Animal Foods*: Despite the commonly held impression that early man was more often a carnivore than an herbivore, recent research has suggested just the reverse. The more likely picture emerging is one of a largely vegetarian humanity. When circumstances have dictated it—in areas of poorer agricultural conditions or more nomadic lifestyles—there has been more reliance on animal sources for protein and fat.

6. *Simple Sugars and Alcohol*: In most regions, the traditional use of milk, fruit, honey and other simple or refined carbohydrate foods have been more as occasional luxury items than as daily staples.[7] Alcohol has functioned in a similar way, occasionally consumed in moderation to help offset the effects of more animal foods or a heavier diet.

This eating pattern has served to support a steady regulation of our metabolism through the generations. As the bulk of our daily food is consumed for energy, complex carbohydrate is the logical choice as a principal food. Simpler sugars tend to bypass the full range of our natural digestive processes, and the "short-cut" way they break down in the body causes us to tire and weaken if consumed in excess. Fats and proteins, on the other hand, have more specialized structural and functional roles, and, if consumed as a primary energy source, place added burdens on our digestion and metabolism, as we will see.

The Changing Modern Diet

"If our great-grandparents spent a day eating with us, they would be wide-eyed and shocked. And if they were plopped down in a modern supermarket, they would probably not know for sure whether they were in a toy, hardware, or grocery store." (From *The Changing American Diet*, Center for Science in the Public Interest, 1978.)

Considering the depth of the whole grain tradition, it is remarkable to realize that in less than a century (in evolutionary terms, the mere blink of an eye) whole cereals as a staple food have all but disappeared from the modern dinner table. The new diet, the diet of modern scientific man, has literally gone against the grain. In fact, our modern diet of the past seventy years represents a radical break from human tradition in almost every respect.

Since the beginning of the century, there has been a progressive decrease in the amount of complex carbohydrates in our diet, and the percentage of carbohydrate supplied by cereal products has fallen well over 50 percent. Furthermore, most of the remaining cereal products that we do eat now consist of refined, often highly processed white breads and similar foods. At the same time, there has been a tremendous increase in consumption of fats, simple sugars, animal proteins, chemicals used in the processing of foods, and animal products in general.[8]

Although the most radical changes in diet have occurred over the past forty years, this shift away from our traditional eating patterns has actually been developing slowly over the past several centuries, largely as a result of the Industrial Revolution and its new technologies and lifestyles. Five major factors can be singled out:

Demographic Changes: Worldwide explorations and new trade routes have introduced foreign food items into regional diets, such as tropical fruits into northern climates, tomatoes and potatoes into European societies and meats into more tropical countries. Together with increasingly active importation, large-scale shifts in population over the past century have brought about the loss of many local dietary traditions.

New Technologies: Nobody knows exactly when the practice of refining grains first began; but over the past several centuries, the Industrial Revolution has ushered in an age of processing, refining, preserving and packaging that has rendered many traditional foods almost unrecognizable.

Affluence: Foods that were once luxury items affordable only to royalty or the rich have become widely available for everyday consumption. These include refined sugar, meats, imported and out-of-season foods, fruit juices and others.

Nutritional Science: The development of the nutritional view of food, while valuable in and of itself, has largely supplanted the wisdom of traditional views on proper dietary practice. For example, many traditions of both hemispheres teach that excessive meat consumption can lead to an overly aggressive character and loss of spiritual sensitivity, yet modern nutritional theory neglects such considerations and views animal products as valuable sources of protein, calcium and iron.

Commerce: Perhaps the most significant factor, food has become a major commodity for mass advertising, which has had a tremendous impact on public choices of what to eat. It is not surprising that those foods that receive virtually no advertising, such as whole grains, fresh vegetables, beans, seeds and fruits, are precisely those that have declined in public favor. The consumption of processed and pre-prepared foods, snack foods, soft drinks, meat and dairy products, on the other hand, have risen in proportion to the marketing efforts mounted to sell them.

It is important to remember that the modern diet was not planned— nobody examined our way of eating at the turn of the century and decided that the diet of 1984 should look as it does today. This historical change has been largely an unplanned experiment, stemming from unprecedented changes in the way we live. The net result has been the loss of our dietary mainstay, whole grains, and a parallel increase in our reliance on items that for thousands of years were luxuries, occasional specialty items or emergency rations.

This radical change has profoundly altered the delicate web of balance within our bodies and with the environment, and particularly in the way we metabolize our foods to release the solar energy they store. To understand the impact of these dietary changes, let us understand the nature of carbohydrates.

Energy and Carbohydrates

Life as we know it would not exist without the *carbon* atom; for it is carbon, the basis of organic chemistry, which is the cornerstone of life's biological alchemy. In plants, carbon acts as a magnet for solar energy, catching the sun's rays with the aid of hydrogen and oxygen and binding them into molecules called *carbohydrates* (also referred to as "saccharides" or "sugars.") The simplest form this energy-binding takes, and the basic building block for all other carbohydrates, is a structure of six carbons and six waters called *glucose* (written as $C_6H_{12}O_6$), a white powder that easily dissolves in water. In order to create more stable forms for storage, plants build these simple glucose molecules into more complex double and multiple sugars, called *disaccharides* and *polysaccharides*.

Double sugars are formed by combining two single sugars (*monosaccharides*) and subtracting one water: $2(C_6H_{12}O_6)-H_2O \rightarrow C_{12}H_{22}O_{10}$. Some common examples are *sucrose* (cane sugar), *maltose* (malt sugar) and *lactose* (milk sugar). Polysaccharides, which include edible *starches* and *cellulose*—the indigestible plant substance that gives plants their rigid "skeleton"—are multiples of a still more stable one-glucose-minus-one-water molecule: $n(C_6H_{10}O_5)$. This is also the formula for *glycogen* or "animal starch," the form glucose takes when we store it in our own bodies. The most common dietary source of energy, starches are abundant in grains, beans, seeds, nuts and many vegetables, while fruits, sugar cane and beet, honey, maple sap and some vegetables are common sources of disaccharide sugar.

Unlike carbohydrate, which is built by stringing together chains of simple glucose molecules, protein is a gigantic, complex and more unstable molecule. It is also composed of carbon, hydrogen and oxygen, with the addition of nitrogen (also abundant in the air you inhale), and often sulphur and phosphorus. Not normally used for fuel, protein's main function is to build and repair body tissues. As our key structural component, protein functions in animals in much the same way cellulose does in plants. Also, many of the body's vital chemical functions are carried out by highly specialized protein molecules, such as enzymes, hormones and vitamins. Fat, unlike both protein and carbohydrate, need only be consumed in very small amounts, as excess dietary carbohydrate can easily be converted to fat in the body. Composed of fairly simple chains of hydrogen and carbon, fat's primary use is as a structural part of nerve, brain and other tissues, and as a fuel reserve. Both protein and fat can be used as fuel when necessary, but this presents some problems, as we shall see.

Once the plant has stored this solar energy, it is ready for us to use. We then harvest, cook, chew and digest it; and in this process, the carbohydrate "knot" is untied by digestive enzymes. The complex chains of starches are gradually reduced to simple glucose, which is then burned as fuel, with the oxygen we breathe fanning the flames. As our glucose is burned, water is given back out through our urination, respiration and perspiration, CO_2 is exhaled, and the sun's energy is released again to animate our existence.

The Importance of Blood Glucose

Without a steady supply of blood glucose (BG) and of oxygen with which to burn it, we would quickly die. And, since the healthy functioning of all our cells depends on their being constantly bathed in this chemically

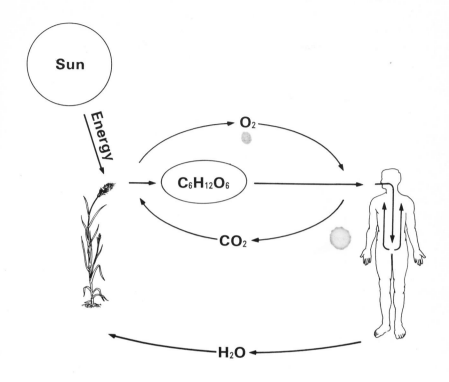

Fig. 4. Plant carbohydrate acts as a storage and transfer medium for introducing solar energy into human circulation, which releases it to our body and brain cells.

stored sunshine, the precise amount of glucose dissolved in the bloodstream is crucial. Too low a level of BG first affects the brain, which uses fully 25 percent of the air you breathe and uses only glucose as its fuel. (Most other tissues can temporarily live off fuels derived from fat.) A moderately glucose deficient bloodstream slowly starves the brain and nervous system, and in particular the cerebral cortex (the seat of conscious thought), producing symptoms of depression, fatigue, nervousness and mental instability. A severely low BG starves all the body's cells and soon leads to coma and death.

At the same time, we cannot handle too much BG all at once. A severe buildup of glucose in the blood rapidly runs the body through a course of weakness, fatigue and again, coma and death, while a chronically but more mildly sugar-rich blood creates a breeding ground for infection, tissue degeneration and other complications, some of them eventually fatal in themselves.

Good health requires that we maintain an extraordinarily steady level of BG at all times; and it is one of nature's miracles that we are able to do just that. The reason we can is that we don't eat glucose itself. If we did, our bloodstream would be at the mercy of our eating habits, and we would need to feed ourselves a steady amount 24 hours a day (the way glucose is fed intravenously in a hospital). Instead, we eat complex sugars, which are simplified only gradually through digestion until they reach the small intestine, where they are steadily fed to the bloodstream at the rate of about two calories per minute. To maintain this steady fire without it's going out every time you fast for a few hours, or flaring up too high every time you eat a large meal, you have a marvelously intricate system of chemical checks and balances to keep the level steady. This system may be called the "glucostat," and functions in much the same way as a thermostat controls a furnace to maintain a steady room temperature.

One way this works is through the conversion of glucose to glycogen (animal starch) and back. When digestion supplies too much glucose to the blood, we can convert the excess into glycogen for storage. Later, when the blood's glucose supply drops too low, that glycogen is retrieved, converted back to glucose, and fed back into the bloodstream.

This process is an example of yin and yang at work. Within the world of plant substances, complex carbohydrate is generally more yang, while the simpler sugars are more yin. The conversion of starch to glucose is a more yin, dissolving process; and any body function which serves to raise the level of blood glucose can be considered to be a more yin process, while lowering the blood glucose is more yang. In the conversion of glucose to glycogen, one water molecule (yin) is removed. Glycogen itself is therefore more yang—for example, it is not water soluble as glucose is—as suits its storage function. The balancing of blood glucose is a beautiful example of yin and yang harmony; and disorders of this balancing can easily be traced to a general imbalance of yin and yang within a whole general condition.

The Functioning of the Glucostat ━━━━━━━━━━

Now let us more closely examine the journey food energy takes as it passes through the body on the way from its stored form in foods to its release as cellular energy. This journey occurs in four general steps.

1. *Absorbing Glucose*, through digestion of food carbohydrates, begins in the mouth as food is chewed. Saliva contains an enzyme called *amylase*

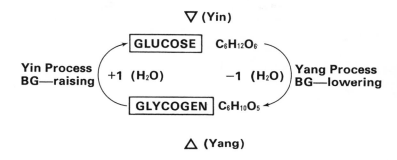

$$\nabla \text{ (Yin)}$$

Yin Process
BG—raising

$+1$ (H_2O)

GLUCOSE $C_6H_{12}O_6$

-1 (H_2O)

GLYCOGEN $C_6H_{10}O_5$

Yang Process
BG—lowering

$$\triangle \text{ (Yang)}$$

Fig. 5. The change from glucose ("blood sugar") to glycogen ("animal starch") and back is accomplished by subtracting and adding a water molecule (yin).

which begins the process of breaking down complex starch chains into simpler forms. This is why repeated chewing of a food high in complex carbohydrate, like carrots, whole wheat bread or brown rice, causes the food to gradually taste sweeter and sweeter. (Cooking, a type of pre-digestion, actually begins this process, which is why a carrot tastes sweeter when cooked than when raw.) Unlike carbohydrate, neither fat nor protein are affected much by the saliva's enzymes. Amylase is mildly alkaline, while protein requires an acid environment for its digestion; and fat generally needs to be acted on by bile before digestion can take place.

After food is swallowed, the stomach begins to secrete digestive juices to further break down its complex structure. After several hours in the stomach, the food enters the duodenum, where a system of ducts (the bile duct, pancreatic duct and common duct joining the two) introduces bile from the gall bladder and digestive fluids from the pancreas, which dissolve the food's structure as it is carried into the small intestine, where the final stages of digestion take place.

Protein's digestion begins in the stomach, and is completed in the duodenum and small intestine. When fat enters the duodenum, it is first *emulsified* (broken into smaller particles) by bile from the liver and gall bladder, and is then digested by pancreatic enzymes.

Carbohydrate is the most yang of these three major nutrients. Protein, being a more delicate, unstable molecule, is more yin; for example, high-protein foods spoil more easily than foods composed largely of starch. Fat is the most yin of the three, as evidenced by the fact that it rises in the presence of water. The body is well designed to balance these differences. The most yin nutrient (fat) is digested in the lowest, or most yang area (the small intestine), while the most yang (carbohydrate) is digested in the uppermost area (the mouth) with protein falling in between in the stomach. This order of nutrients is also reflected in their order of digestion—the most yang, carbohydrate, digests first, while the most yin, fat, is the slowest to digest. The presence of both protein and particularly fat slow down digestion in the stomach, while a less "rich" meal of mostly carbohydrates proceeds more quickly, being digested mainly in the mouth and small intestine. Protein and fat, then, are nutritional "specialty" items, supplying vital special functions to the body, but only at the expense of a slightly heavier digestive burden, and they are traditionally eaten in much smaller volume than carbohydrates.

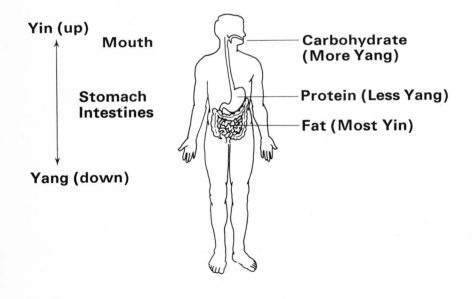

Fig. 6. The body is designed to digest the most yin macronutrient (fat) in the most yang (lowest) area, and the most yang macronutrient (complex carbohydrate) in the most yin (highest) area.

The digestion of simple and refined sugar also differs from that of complex carbohydrates. The action of salivary amylase tends to be inhibited by simple sugars, which can also interfere with the digestion of starches if they are both eaten together. Further, since the molecules of simple sugars are so small, they often bypass the lengthy starch-splitting digestive process, and pass directly into the bloodstream through the walls of the mouth or stomach. Alcohol, some drugs and some spices or flavoring agents also have this quick-entering ability. Simple sugar and these other items are also much more yin than complex carbohydrate.

Up to this point, your food is technically considered as being still "outside" your body. In the small intestine, after the foods have been reduced to their most basic components (glucose, amino acids, fatty acids and others), they are finally absorbed through the intestinal wall into tiny blood capillaries, and enter the bloodstream. It is at this point that food is considered as being "inside" you. This newly nutrient-rich blood is now gathered and delivered up through the portal vein to the liver, which masterminds its use. The liver may filter out various impurities (such as chemical pollutants, drugs or other toxins), alter the chemical or hormonal content of the blood, put part of it into storage, or change it in a number of other ways before it is finally sent to the heart and put into circulation. One of the important functions that happens here in the liver is that the BG level of this new blood is carefully measured and, if need be, altered.

2. *Storing Excess Glucose.* The amount of blood glucose needed for proper metabolism is about 100 mg per 100 cc of blood (usually written as 100 mg percent. As your food is slowly being digested and absorbed, th ımount may trickle steadily into the portal vein's new blood. However, if you have eaten a particularly large meal, or if your meal contained a large load of simple sugars that were absorbed more quickly, you soon exceed acceptable BG limits, and some of that excess glucose needs to be taken out of circulation. This is accomplished in two ways.

First, some of that glucose is delivered to the body's cells to be burned as fuel; vigorous exercise (yang) will bring the blood glucose level down. If there is still excess left over, the liver begins to change it into glycogen in a process called *glycogenesis.* Glycogen, once formed, is stored in the liver itself and in the body's muscles, ready to be taken out of storage again when needed.

After the body's capacity to store glycogen is exceeded (which happens fairly readily), or if the glycogenesis process doesn't proceed smoothly due to an overburdening or weakness of the liver, excess glucose may be delivered to fat cells and converted to *triglycerides*, a storage form of fat. When relied upon regularly however, this process results in obesity. Storage of energy as glycogen is more yang, and as triglycerides, more yin.

3. *Energy Retrieval.* Long after the meal is done, when the supplies of new glucose from the intestines have been exhausted, the BG begins to dip too low. This signals the liver and other organs to begin calling some of those reserves back into circulation. Glycogen is pulled out of storage and changed back into glucose (made more yin) by the addition of a water molecule (*glycohydrolisis*). However, between the liver, with a glucogen-storing capacity of about 70 gm, and the muscles, which on the average can store another 200–400 gm, and free glucose available in various body fluids (only about 15–20 gm), there is only enough stored glucose available for a maximum of one day's energy needs.[9] Depending on an individual's size, there may up to three months' energy supply stored as fat; but fat is not a preferred fuel. Once glycogen stores are exhausted, then, the low BG level triggers the sensation of hunger to bring in new sources of glucose. If no new food is eaten, a fourth process steps into action.

4. *Creation of New Energy Fuels.* When your body's glycogen stores have been depleted, or if for some reason the glycogen-to-glucose conversion process is not operating smoothly (which is sometimes the case), your muscles begin to release their *amino acids* (protein's primary component) into the bloodstream, which are delivered to the liver and converted to glucose. This process, called *gluconeogenesis*, creates some new problems however. First, the nitrogen in proteins is left over to form various waste products (principally urea), which add to the body's excretory burden. Excess urea, for example, can crystallize as the uric acid deposits of gout. Second, and more important, the amino acids pulled into circulation for energy can't be used to rebuild damaged tissues or build muscles. If this continues for long, the muscles begin to waste away and the body's structure begins to break down. To avoid this destructive process, gluconeogensis is provided with a back-up system that utilizes fats.

Your body's fat reserves are now pulled out of storage, again to the liver, and are converted to fuel. Fats are not changed to glucose, but are split into their components *glycerol* and *fatty acids*. Glycerol is then easily converted into glucose and burned; but the bulk of fat, the fatty acids, are used as fuel without being changed to glucose. Once again, however, this process causes problems of its own. First, fatty acids cannot be completely burned, and are therefore not a "clean" fuel as is carbohydrate. When burned in the presence of carbohydrate, the combustion of fats is somewhat cleaner; but in the absence of glucose, a great deal of *diacetic acid* and *acetone* are left.[10] A moderate amount of these toxins can be temporarily "buffered" or neutralized by the body's mineral reserves; but a sizable buildup of these blood acids will eventually deplete your minerals and lead to a condition of *acidosis,* causing you to become drowsy, weak, and finally comatose. This is why prolonged fasting and starvation, which causes one to draw on fat reserves as fuel, can cause severe acidosis and coma. Figure 7 illustrates the balancing of yin and yang this process maintains.

Since the process of manufacturing emergency fuels is clearly a stop gap measure with potentially harmful side-effects, only a diet high in complex carbohydrates can adequately maintain a steady BG level without undue strain. As long as our way of eating relies on whole grains and the other moderate, traditional staples, we can easily manage the small adjustments needed to keep this balance. But as we have abandoned whole grains and come to rely far more heavily on foods with more extreme yin or yang tendencies and higher fat, protein and simple sugar contents, this natural balance has become disrupted. As a result, the majority of us have gradually developed chronic patterns of imbalanced or widely fluctuating blood glucose metabolism; namely diabetes and hypoglycemia.

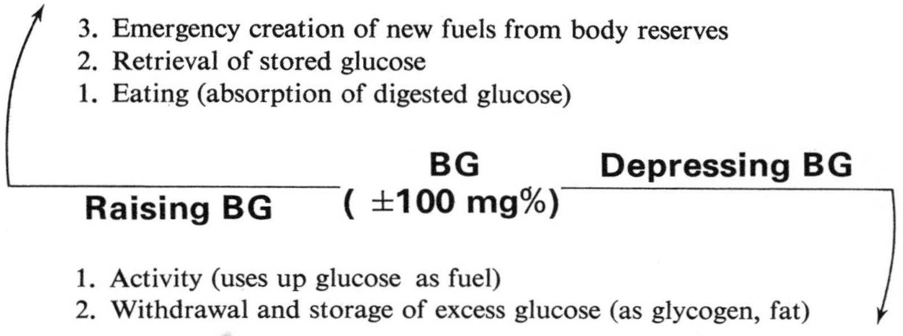

3. Emergency creation of new fuels from body reserves
2. Retrieval of stored glucose
1. Eating (absorption of digested glucose)

BG   **Depressing BG**

Raising BG   **(±100 mg%)**

1. Activity (uses up glucose as fuel)
2. Withdrawal and storage of excess glucose (as glycogen, fat)

Fig. 7. The "glucostat": functions by balancing the level of blood glucose (BG).

The Progressive Development of Sickness ───────────

To understand how sickness develops, we can compare the human form to that of a tree. A tree's sustenance comes from the nutrients absorbed from the soil through the tree's roots, creating sap which is distributed to the trunk, branches and ultimately, the leaves and fruits. If the quality of nourishment in the soil is chronically poor, the final result (the fruits and leaves) begin to lose their ability to function normally and gradually deteriorate.

In the human form, it is the quality of our food, absorbed through our intestinal "roots" that creates the quality of our blood (our "sap") and determines the health or sickness of all our cells, tissues and organs. By the time obvious symptoms of illness actually appear on the surface, an unhealthy inner condition of the blood has usually been already in progress for a long time, perhaps even decades. (In the case of children who become seriously ill, it is generally the parents' way of eating and blood quality that has laid the basis for sickness.) In other words, major sicknesses never arise suddenly; they are the more advanced stages of a long-term process.

Normally we are able to discharge unhealthy excesses from extreme dietary habits through the channels of urination, bowel movement, respiration, perspiration, activity (caloric discharge) and others. In more extreme instances, we may mobilize this discharging ability through unusual behaviors such as sneezing, trembling, fevers, skin rashes, or extreme emotions and expression, to eliminate built-up excesses and return to a healthy equilibrium. Eventually, however, if we continue to maintain an immoderate diet, these toxic buildups begin to accumulate at different sites in the body's interior, often in the form of mucus and fat deposits, stones, cysts and tumors. Depending on the particular location of these accumulations, different organs and functions are affected, and the process may finally lead to their impairment or degeneration.[11]

Even in the earlier stages, this process naturally puts a progressively greater strain on the glucostat system (among other metabolic functions). As excesses begin to stagnate about the glands and organs responsible for keeping the BG steady, the problem worsens and becomes chronic, and in some cases, even degenerative. Let us look at the glands and organs that are affected in this case.

Carbohydrate Metabolism and Hormones ───────────

The term *metabolism* refers to all the changes in energy and materials that build, repair and fuel our bodies. All the complex processes of metabolism are controlled by two opposing, balancing functions referred to as anabolism and catabolism, which reflect the energies of yin and yang. *Anabolism* is a yang, constructive force, including the building of tissues out of free materials available in the circulation, while its opposite *catabolism* is a yin, destructive force which takes apart tissues and returns their materials into free circulation. Putting glucose into storage, introducing circulating glucose into a cell where it is burned as fuel, and storing excess glucose as fat, are all anabolic and represent more yang energies. Reducing complex carbohydrate to glucose through digestion, changing stored glycogen back to glucose, and creating new fuels by releasing muscular protein or fat into circulation are all more yin, catabolic functions.

These operations are commandeered by the ductless or *endocrine glands*, which are those glands in the body that manufacture highly specialized and powerful fluids called *hormones* and release them directly into the bloodstream. The endocrine glands that have key roles in glucose metabolism are the *pancreas*, which lies on the left side behind the stomach, the *adrenal glands*, which sit atop each kidney on the right and left sides, and to a lesser extent, the *thyroid*, *pituitary* and *gonads* (the ovaries and testes). The liver itself and tiny glands embedded in the intestines also play important roles in this process.

When in good health, the pancreas has a rich, golden-yellow color, though in sickness and upon autopsy its radiant sheen fades to a withered straw-yellow. Somewhat resembling a fish in shape, it measures about eight inches from head to tail; its head is nestled at the center of the torso (the *solar plexus*) against the curve of the duodenum, its body and tail extending upward and to the left.

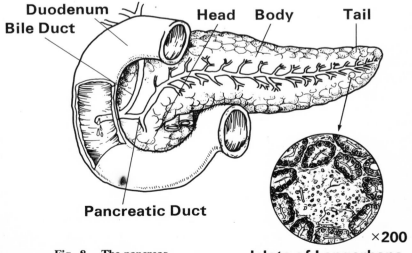

Duodenum
Bile Duct
Head Body Tail
Pancreatic Duct
×200
Fig. 8. The pancreas.
Islets of Langerhans

The hollow *pancreatic duct* runs from left to right, collecting the pancreas's digestive secretions and depositing them together with bile from the liver into the duodenum. (This digestive function of the pancreas is unrelated to its endocrine function.) Scattered through the tissue surrounding the central duct are irregularly shaped cords of cells, called the *Islets of Langerhans*. These are most numerous in the tail, and consist of four cell types: A cells, B cells, D cells and F cells (the first three are also called alpha, beta and delta). Each cell type secretes its own hormone(s) which do not enter the duct, but pass directly into the body's general blood circulation through tiny capillaries permeating the gland's tissue.

- The B or beta cells secrete *insulin*, the hormone so well-known in connection with diabetes. Insulin literally means "islet hormone."
- The A or alpha cells secrete *glucagon* or "anti-insulin," which opposes the action of insulin and is also thought to have a role in diabetes. It is also used as an injected antidote to counteract an accidental overdose of injected insulin.
- The D or delta cells secrete two more hormones that control secretions of the first two: *somatostatin*, which inhibits the secretion of both alpha and beta cells, and *gastrin*, which has the opposite effect.
- The F cells secrete *pancreatic polypeptide*, which is thought to help regulate the entire balance of both endocrine and exocrine (digestive) functions of the pancreas and the stomach as well.

Insulin

In the control of glucose metabolism, insulin is the only hormone that has a yang, anabolic effect. Insulin lowers the BG by causing free circulating glucose to be introduced into body cells and burned as fuel. Without the presence of insulin, most tissues cannot use this glucose for fuel. Insulin is like the "key" that unlocks the cell's door to allow glucose to enter. It also lowers BG by promoting glycogenesis and inhibiting glycogenolysis; that is, helping glucose to change into glycogen, and keep it from changing back to glucose. Further, it can lower BG by inhibiting the creation of new glucose fuels, or gluconeogenesis.

Insulin also causes amino acids to enter muscles and build protein, and causes sugar and free fatty acids to enter fat cells and be stored as new fat (*lipogenesis*). At the same time, insulin inhibits the opposite from happening: it prevents the breakdown of protein and fat into their components. And finally, although this does not relate so directly to carbohydrate metabolism, insulin is the major hormone responsible for the prodigious growth of a fetus during gestation.[12] This demonstrates what a powerfully anabolic or "body-building" substance insulin is!

A brief review of the characteristics of yin and yang reveals that all of these functions are more yang, producing a gathering, building or glucose-lowering effect. Insulin itself, therefore, can be classified as a yang hormone. Interestingly, the insulin-secreting beta cells are most numerous in the more dense, yang central portion of the pancreas's tail, while the more yin alpha cells appear more toward the surface.

Insulin-Opposing Hormones

Counteracting the action of insulin are a number of more yin hormones that have the effect of raising the BG level. Since they work counter to insulin, these are called "counter-regulatory" hormones; and all of them can be considered catabolic.

- Glucagon, secreted by the more yin alpha cells, is also referred to as "anti-insulin." The presence of digestive activity in the small intestine stimulates the secretion of glucagon, which in turn stimulates the release of glucose and fatty acids into the bloodstream. Normally, high levels of glucagon in the blood stimulates the release of more insulin, so the rise in BG doesn't get out of hand.[13]
- The adrenal glands secrete a variety of BG-raising hormones. The first group, secreted by the adrenal *cortex*, or outer portion, are called *adreno-cortical* hormones, and are responsive to mild stress conditions. Those that affect glucose metabolism are called *gluco-corticoids*, and these are the hormones that are normally brought into play to restore balance when BG dips slightly too low.
- The front part of the pituitary gland secretes a hormone called *ACTH*, for *adreno-corticotropic hormone*, which literally means what is does: stimulates the production of hormones from the adrenal cortex (above). (While this front or "anterior" region of the pituitary is more yin, the posterior area is more yang and secretes *vasopressin*, an anti-diuretic hormone, and *oxytocin*, which causes the contractions of childbirth.)
- *Enteric* hormones, secreted by tiny glands in the stomach and intestine, are stimulated by the mere presence of food in the digestive tract. These all raise the BG level.[14]
- *Thyroxin*, secreted by the thyroid gland, also further stimulates the action of the adrenals, and like ACTH, has the effect of raising BG.
- Finally, under emergency circumstances the inner or *medulla* portion of the adrenals are signaled to secrete *epinephrine*, better known as *adrenaline*, which is the "fight or flight" hormone we have all felt

the effects of when under stress. Its effects are to raise the BG, speed the pulse, sharpen the senses, and generally key up the organism for sharper functioning when under duress.

Working together, the mild action of the enteric hormones and glucagon, corrective action of the adrenal cortex and the occasional emergency boost provided by adrenaline, all serve to balance insulin's BG-lowering effect. Each hormone's deployment is tied to all the others, and the body is normally kept from going too far in one direction or the other. That, however, is exactly what does happen in diabetes and hypoglycemia.

The Development of Diabetes and Hypoglycemia

A recent series of studies has revealed an interesting pattern. Women who are obese primarily in the upper body are eight times more prone to diabetes than normal or lower-body-obese women.[15] There is also an anatomical distinction between the two types of obesity. Lower body obese women have increased numbers of normal sized fat cells, while upper body obese women have normal numbers of enlarged fat cells.

This is a marvelous illustration of yin and yang. Upper body fat is the result of more yin dietary excesses such as sugar, milk and soft dairy foods, and refined foods, while lower body fat is caused more by overconsumption of eggs, meats and more salty, denser dairy products such as hard cheeses. While the increased numbers of fat cells in the lower body is an yin symptom (fat in general being yin), the increased size of upper body fat cells is far more expanded and yin. Not surprisingly, the study also revealed that the lower body fat (more yang) is much harder to lose —that is, it is more yang, stubborn and tenacious—while the upper body, more yin, superficial fat can be shed far more easily.

YIN	YANG
upper body fat	lower body fat
larger fat cells	greater numbers of fat cells
easier to lose	harder to lose
cause: milk, sugar, etc.	cause: eggs, cheeses, etc.
more commonly diabetic	more rarely diabetic

This clue alone would suggest that diabetes is a disease caused by more yin extremes; and this proves to be exactly the case. As a result of chronic overconsumption of sugar, sweetened foods, milk and dairy products, refined flour and other more yin foods, the blood glucose is continually

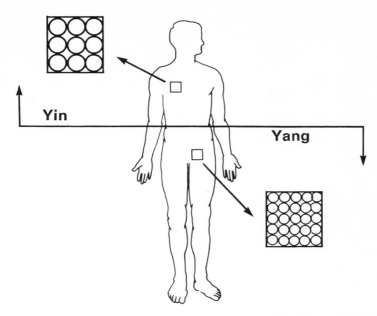

Fig. 9. Fat cell biopsies reveal a different composition of upper body fat (yin) and lower body fat (yang) in women. Upper-obese women are eight times more prone to diabetes (yin).

pushed upward (yin) until eventually the system is unable to bring the BG down into normal ranges at all. As an extreme expression of this yin nature, the cell clusters of the pancreas actually begin to decompose, with degeneration then spreading throughout the body to affect many other locations.

As the pancreas and other glands begin to weaken, the yang hormone insulin is either not produced, underproduced, or not used effectively. Without the body-building, anabolic effects of insulin, the body is soon in a state of crisis.

1. In the absence of insulin, glucose will not enter most body cells to be burned as fuel; and it will not be stored in the liver or muscles as glycogen. Free glucose therefore begins to build up in the bloodstream, while most of the body's cells begin to starve for energy.

2. In the absence of insulin's control, all the body's BG-raising functions continue unchecked. Any stores of glycogen will be reconverted to glucose, absorption of glucose from the gut will be constantly stimulated, and the conversion of glycerol and amino acids to glucose will step up their pace. This increasing supply of glucose

isn't utilized as fuel, but simply builds up in the blood.

3. At the same time, without insulin's inhibiting effect, the catabolic breakdown of muscle protein and body fat accelerates, while the rebuilding of muscle and fat tissues cannot take place. This results in a deterioration of the muscles, weight loss, and general weakness and wasting of the body. At the same time, the bloodstream becomes flooded with amino acids and free fatty substances.

4. When the concentration of BG reaches a dangerous level, the kidneys step into action as an escape valve and remove the excess, passing it out of the body dissolved in urine. This "renal threshold" is about 180 mg percent. *Glycosuria* (glucose in the urine) and *polyuria* (profuse urination) are the most well-known and often the most obvious symptoms of diabetes. Since this results in a tremendous loss of water (up to 15 percent of total body weight may be lost in urination[16]), it is accompanied by tremendous thirst (*polydipsia*), as well as the profound hunger associated with the loss of protein and weight. Unfortunately, the loss of fluid makes the blood more concentrated, raising still further the concentration of sugar in the blood.

5. The buildup of fat in the blood puts a tremendous strain on the liver, which tries to neutralize excess fat; and the blood's acidity begins to rise dangerously. To buffer this, mineral reserves are called upon, further depleting the body's strength. Eventually the production of acetone and ketoacids reaches an uncontrollable level. The condition of *ketoacidosis*, unique to diabetics, is the fatal result.

Hypoglycemia ("hypo" means too little and "glycemia" refers to glucose) is a condition opposite to that of diabetes: Yang insulin secretion becomes overly powerful, or the more yin functions that oppose insulin grow stagnated and weakened, producing a deficiency of circulating blood glucose. Hypoglycemia is more typically a disorder of gathering, stagnating accumulation rather than of degeneration and decomposition, revealing its more yang, concentrating nature. The same types of foods that cause lower body obesity, particularly animal foods and salt, begin to gather around the compact, dense glands and organs responsible for keeping the blood glucose level from dropping too low. Frequently the hypoglycemic person begins to respond to this developing condition reflexively by relying on strongly yin items such as coffee, sugared foods, alcohol or drugs; but rather than erasing the accumulations of overly yang foods, this only serves to aggravate the high and low swings of blood glucose, with a correspondingly chaotic pattern of mood and personality changes.

Fig. 10. The lack of complex carbohydrates such as whole grains makes the BG-balancing system unstable; depending upon the more yin or more yang nature of foods used, diabetes or hypoglycemia may result.

Hypoglycemia (more △)	Diabetes (more ▽)
Eggs	Tropical fruits and vegetables
Poultry	Milk, dairy products
Cheeses, salty dairy foods	Oil and oily foods
Meats	Refined flour products
Overly salty foods	Sweetened beverages (juices, soft drinks)
Oily, greasy foods	In some cases, drugs and medications

PLUS

Refined sugar, sweets
Refined flour
Tropical fruit juices
Soft drinks, alcohol
In some cases, drugs and medications

In rare cases, the lack of glucose in the blood can starve the nervous system to the point of coma and death within days or even hours. Far more commonly, though, is the milder condition of a chronically subnormal blood glucose, often referred to as *functional hypoglycemia.* This generally produces the following effects:

1. Not surprisingly, the low glucose level can stimulate a ravenous hunger (commonly considered a yang symptom); hypoglycemia is sometimes referred to as the "hunger disease." However, since normal eating doesn't bring the BG level up to where it should be, this voracious appetite isn't satisfied. Following the law that yang attracts yin, the person will often be attracted to concentrated, simple sugars in an effort to force the BG up, only to experience a "crash" within several hours as the overstimulated insulin functions bring the BG plummeting down again. Coffee, which "whips" the adrenals into action, alcohol and other drugs may become habitual; but the higher the "highs" are, the more vigorously the body's unbalanced system brings new downs.

2. Continuing lack of glucose stimulates an adrenaline reaction; a milder reaction produces a general buildup of internal stress and fatigue, as the body is on a constant or chronic "alert." The more extreme adrenaline reaction produces a condition of intense nervousness, heart palpitations, chills and sometimes nausea.

3. Never falling too low to be acutely dangerous, the chronic dips in blood glucose primarily affect the brain, which begins to starve constantly for glucose. (Remember that other body tissues can survive on amino acids, glycerol and fatty acids, but the brain requires glucose for its functioning, and particularly the cerebral cortex.) This results in a constant feeling of depression, anxiety, neurosis or other personality changes.

4. The combination of constant internal stress, glucose starvation to the cells, and the excessive buildup of fat and protein tissue brought about by the unchecked flow of insulin, often lead to more localized secondary disorders such as asthma, allergies, glandular exhaustion or psychiatric problems.

Early Detection and Prevention —————————————————

It is possible to detect the beginnings of these disorders well before the chronic or degenerative stages have developed, and to prevent the process from continuing by adopting a more moderate diet. Even the most advanced stages of either problem can almost always be improved by making such a change; but the earlier the change is made, the greater the possibility for fully recovering normal health.

This "early detection" is possible because internal conditions also appear in various external regions, such as in the face, eyes and limbs. In the case of hypoglycemia, the pancreas, liver and adrenal glands are especially affected, while a tendency toward diabetes can often be seen by observing traits that correspond to ill health in the pancreas, large intestine, lungs and spleen. Figure 11 shows some of the common signs of these tendencies. Additional possible signs of either tendency include distortion or twisting of the large toe on either foot. (This last arises because the acupuncture meridians leading to and from the pancreas and liver terminate in these toes.)[17]

Diabetes and Hypoglycemia: Complementary Opposites

When diabetes progresses to the point of ketoacidosis, the body is thrown into an acute yin condition known as *diabetic coma*. The opposite, more acutely yang condition is called *insulin shock*, a state of profound hypoglycemia most commonly induced by an accidental overdose of insulin. Reviewing the symptoms of these two opposite states provides another illustration of the yin and yang nature of the two disorders. For example, the intense anxiety and confusion, pounding heartbeat, headache and rapidity of onset of hypoglycemic (insulin) shock are all more yang

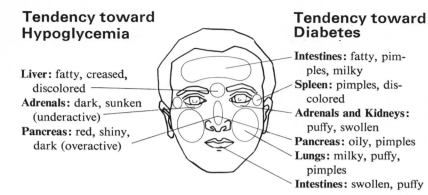

Tendency toward Hypoglycemia

Liver: fatty, creased, discolored
Adrenals: dark, sunken (underactive)
Pancreas: red, shiny, dark (overactive)

Tendency toward Diabetes

Intestines: fatty, pimples, milky
Spleen: pimples, discolored
Adrenals and Kidneys: puffy, swollen
Pancreas: oily, pimples
Lungs: milky, puffy, pimples
Intestines: swollen, puffy

Fig. 11. Different facial characteristics often reveal internal conditions that may show a tendency toward blood sugar imbalances.

symptoms, as compared to the more yin symptoms characterizing diabetic coma, including lethargy, labored breathing, excessive urination, a weak pulse and a slow, gradual onset.

Insulin Shock (yang)	Symptom	Diabetic Coma (yin)
sudden, rapid	onset	slow, gradual
intense anxiety & confusion	mental state	lethargy, slurred or incoherent speech
pounding, rapid	pulse	rapid, weak
strong hunger, nausea	appetite	no hunger, extreme thirst
headache & dizziness	headache	none
shallow breathing	breath	heavy, labored breathing, acetone odor
moist	tongue	dry
pale, clammy	skin	hot, dry, often flushed
normal or less	urination	profuse urination with sweet or acetone odor

Ironically, while these two conditions represent extreme opposites, they are often confused with each other (and either is commonly mistaken for an alcoholic or drug-induced stupor.) It is vitally important to be able to distinguish between the two, since administering the wrong treatment can easily prove fatal. An injection of insulin is needed to recover from diabetic coma. Hypoglycemic shock or insulin overdose should be treated with a concentrated source of carbohydrate, such as fruit juice or a concentrated sweetener dissolved in water or placed under the tongue. (In very mild cases of insulin-induced hypoglycemia it may be enough to eat a handful of nuts or crackers, while in severe cases resulting in unconsciousness, an injection of glucagon may be needed.)

In summary, diabetes is a yin, over-catabolic condition, and hypoglycemia a yang, over-anabolic state. For centuries, we have maintained a productive harmony with the environment, our lives centered around the tilling of soil and developing the richness of culture reaped from its harvests. Through a carefully balanced way of eating centered on whole cereals and vegetables, we have delivered the sun's stored energies to each of our body's cells in a consistently harmonious way commensurate with our traditionally moderate lifestyle. Our modern way of eating has lost that stabilizing influence and given way to extremes, in the process losing the dietary thread through the labyrinth of our glucose metabolism. In effect, we may say that the sun shines too bright in the diabetic's bloodstream, and he is consumed in its brilliant flames or smoldering embers. The hypoglycemic, on the contrary, is in an internal state of perpetual twilight, the body's and brain's cells never receiving the normally full exposure to that internal sunshine, creating a pervasive feeling of darkness, pessimism or gloom, and a sense of constant struggle. In both cases, the central issue in preventing or recovering from either disorder is the reestablishment of an orderly, balanced continuity with our environment, through the medium of our daily food.

---

[1]   These and other general statistics in this volume, where not quoted directly, are compiled from a variety of sources listed in the bibliography.

[2]   Light (*Hypoglycemia: One of Man's Most Widespread and Misdiagnosed Diseases*, Marilyn Light, listed in bibliography), p. 1. References from sources listed in the bibliography are entered below under author's last name.

[3]   Light, p. 21, and cf. Dufty, p. 91 ff.

[4]   For a more complete discussion of yin and yang, please refer to *The Cancer Prevention Diet, The Book of Macrobiotics, Natural Healing Through Macrobiotics*, and other works by the author.

[5]   Ballantine, p. 280 ff.

[6]   For more discussion of biological evolution and its impact on human diet, please refer to *The Book of Macrobiotics*.

[7]   Ballantine, op cit.

[8]   For more detail on these dietary changes, please refer to *The Changing American Diet* and *Dietary Goals for the United States*.

[9]   1 gram of glucose provides about 4 kcal; 1 kcal fuels about 1 minute of the body's "basal metabolism" or minimum activities.

[10]   Abrahamson, p. 22.

[11]   This progression is described in more detail in the author's *Cancer Prevention Diet*, pp. 35–41 and *Natural Healing Through Macrobiotics*, pp. 23–33.

[12]   Brothers, p. 54.

[13]   For reference to this and the following hormones' roles, cf. Bernstein, p. 39 ff.

[14]   They are called enteroglucagon, secretin, somatostatin, gastrin, cholecystokinin and GIP, or Gastric Inhibitory Polypeptide.

[15]   "A New Marker for Diabetes," *Science*, Vol. 215, Feb. 5, 1982, p. 651.

[16]   Brothers, p. 23.

[17]   For more on traditional and macrobiotic methods of diagnosis, please refer to *How to See Your Health* and *Your Face Never Lies*.

2. Diabetes

"Five million Americans have diabetes and don't know it," ran the headline of a recent ad for a prominent producer of commercial insulin; yet even this shocking figure may actually be understating the case. According to the most commonly accepted estimates, *diabetes mellitus* or "sugar diabetes" affects eleven million Americans, roughly 5 percent of the population, and costs the nation a staggering $15.7 billion per year. 25 percent of the population has either diabetes or a diabetic relative, and every fifth American baby born this year is expected to have the disease within his or her lifetime. Diabetes is the leading cause of new blindness, kidney failure and gangrene resulting in amputation of the legs. It reduces life expectancy by 33 percent, and is one of the prime causes of heart and vascular diseases. Those particularly at rick for diabetes, though the disease may strike within any population group, are the overweight and the elderly—the likelihood of getting diabetes doubles with each decade of life and every 20 percent of additional excess body weight—and the poor, particularly within affluent nations. Though global in scope, with an estimated worldwide incidence of 300 million (America accounts for only 1/30 of the Earth's diabetic population), the prevalence of diabetes is especially high in the more affluent nations, where overconsumption of a more modernized, less traditional diet is more common.

However, these figures may tell only part of the story. There are 5.5 million diagnosed diabetics, with estimates of another 5.5 million undiagnosed cases. Some experts believe, though, that there may actually be three to four times that number of undiagnosed diabetics—up to 20 million in the U.S. (10 percent of the population), and up to 1.2 billion worldwide![1] It is suspected, for example, that the rate of undetected diabetes in victims of cardiovascular disease is much higher than usually stated. Spot-check blood tests on elderly in nursing homes have yielded diabetic level diagnoses of nearly 100 percent![2] In 1977, the US Department of Health, Education and Welfare reported that data may seriously underestimate diabetes' contribution to mortality. The disease itself was coded as the cause of death in only 26 percent of all diabetics, and actually appeared on only 10 percent of diagnosed diabetics' death certificates. Finally, the costs cited above don't include expenses related to diabetic complications, which are actually the cause of death in six out of seven cases recorded. In any case, and by any definition, diabetes is a twentieth century epidemic, and one which, unlike heart disease, has shown no signs of slowing its alarming rate of increase.

Curiously, the public is not generally aware of the scope or dangers of the problem; and this contributes to the insidious nature of the disease. We are intimately knowledgeable about our Number One cause of death, cardiovascular illness; and the current Number Two killer, cancer, is the disease Americans fear most. Yet how many know, for example, that one half of all heart disease deaths are caused by diabetes? Those who do know about diabetes usually think it can be cured, or at least well controlled, with insulin or oral medications—and in the words of one authority, "nothing could be further from the truth."[3]

Despite the tremendous intensity of the diabetes research effort in this century, and the formidable amount of knowledge concerning many of the minute details of the disease, there is still no agreement in scientific circles as to what causes diabetes. In fact, even the history of the disorder is shrouded in mystery and misconception: and in seeking to unravel some of the puzzles of diabetes, a brief look at this history should prove illustrative.

Diabetes Mellitus: Ancient or Modern? ━━━━━━━

One of the oldest known medical documents, the Ebers Papyrus (dating from about 1500 B.C.), contains a number of prescriptions for "medicines to drive away the passing of too much urine."[4] Since polyuria is one of the most obvious symptoms of diabetes, it has long been thought that the disease was well-known to the Western world as early as 3,500 years ago. Seventeen hundred years later, the noted physician Aretaeus in Alexandria described a "rare" disease characterized by polyuria, in which "the fluid uses the patient's body as a ladder to escape downwards." He cited the Greek word diabaiton, meaning "ladder," as the origin of the term diabetes. Historians are still unclear on the original derivation of the word; it may also have stemmed from words meaning "standing with the legs apart," or "syphon." In any case, it seems clear that profuse urination was the outstanding symptom from the beginning.

However, there are two other symptoms that can hardly be missed even by casual observation. First, owing to the unusual presence of glucose, the diabetic's urine has an exceptionally sweet taste and smell. Until the development of modern methods for testing the urine chemically, a common practice for diagnosing diabetes was to actually taste the urine. In fact, this practice, called *urinoscopy*, was in common use from 400 B.C. until A.D. 1600[5]—yet there is no description in the annals of Western medicine of this sweet urine.

Further, due to the elevated levels of acetone in the diabetic's blood, an unmistakable odor of acetone appears on the breath at the onset of keto-acidosis. Doctors monitoring the diabetic wards in early hospitals routinely sniffed each patient's breath to detect this odor (which resembles the smell of new-mown hay). Yet again, there is no mention of this obvious symptom in any records prior to the 1600's.

In fact, there is considerable doubt as to whether "sugar diabetes" was observed at all in any of these early records. Galen, the greatest medical authority in the Roman empire, used the term diabetes and recorded a total of two cases; yet he doesn't mention the telltale acetone breath or sweet urine. A South African expert on diabetes, Dr. G. D. Campbell, has declared,

"I find it hard to explain why Hippocrates never described a case of diabetes. Such a careful clinical observer could hardly have failed to recognize its florid manifestations, either alone or complicating one of the many cases [of other illnesses] that he meticulously described."[6]

The medical historian Henschen offers a plausible explanation for this puzzle: there is a rare type of diabetes called *diabetes insipidus*, in which the lack of a natural anti-diuretic hormone called vasopressin produces excessive urination and thirst.[7] This disorder, however, has nothing whatsoever to do with glucose metabolism; there is no sugar in the urine, no acetone on the breath, no ketoacidosis, and none of the other complications of diabetes mellitus. (In this volume, the term "diabetes" refers exclusively to diabetes mellitus, also known popularly as "sugar diabetes," unless otherwise noted.) In all likelihood, then, the well-known diabetes we are discussing here had its first appearance in the Western hemisphere in the 1600's, when the term "mellitus" (meaning "honey-sweet") was first coined.

In the Far East, however, the earliest unambiguous records of diabetes mellitus appear to have emerged about 1,000 years earlier than in the West. The venerated Chinese medical text *Nei Ching*, the *Yellow Emperor's Classic of Internal Medicine*, refers to a condition called *xiao-ke*, literally "wasting and thirsting."[8] Though it is unclear whether or not this actually refers to diabetes (it, too, may describe diabetes insipidus), it is at least clear that by the seventh century A.D. Chinese physicians were describing the sweet urine of diabetes mellitus. Trowell claims that the disease was known for at least 2,000 years in India, where it was considered as a problem found mainly among the wealthy and immoderate.[9] Charaka, an Indian physician writing circa A.D. 150, describes *madhumeh* (honey urine) as a common disease. Again, according to Trowell:

"Obesity and diabetes mellitus . . . usually emerge together about the same time in any community that is becoming affluent, wherein the wealthy are able to consume more fat, oil, sugar, meat, wine and beer, also refined cereals, such as white bread and white rice. Little is known concerning the ancient date when, in India and China, rice began to be [processed] to produce low fibre white rice . . . . Perhaps this explains why diabetes mellitus emerges as a common disease at an early date [compared with the Western world] in India and China."[10]

From the standpoint of yin and yang, it is easy to see why this difference between East and West should arise. The diet of the Orient has traditionally relied far less on animal foods, and can generally be classified as more yin. In the West, poorer agricultural conditions and more active, migratory lifestyles have produced a more yang diet with more animal foods, more salt and less variety or quantity of yin foods. For example, sugar, tea, coffee and spices were all introduced to the West from the Orient, while the practice of regularly consuming beef has been introduced only recently in countries such as India and Japan.

These differences in diet have produced a tendency towards more non-aggressive, reflective, spiritually motivated cultures in the East, as well as more susceptibility to a yin disease such as diabetes. In the West they have resulted in more aggressive, active and technologically innovative cultures with more of a tendency toward yang disorders such as hypoglycemia.

The Emergence of Diabetes in Europe

The European appearance of diabetes during the seventeenth century was related to two significant developments: obesity as a common condition, and the widespread consumption of refined sugar. Obesity was an uncommon condition in the English upper social classes until the eighteenth century, shortly after the first appearance of diabetes. Trowell states that diabetes and obesity appear together "and the prevalence increases, about the same period of time and always in upper social groups";[11] and indeed, it was the physician to the English royalty, Sir Thomas Willis, who first described diabetes in 1674.[12] Since Aretaeus's work had recently received its first publication in Latin (1552), Willis borrowed the term diabetes and added "mellitus," the Latin for "honeyed," to describe the new disease.

Obesity, in turn, has been firmly linked with the overconsumption of refined foods, and particularly refined sugar, in population studies conducted throughout the world. By 1662, annual sugar consumption in England had increased from virtually zero to about sixteen million pounds, all in less than two centuries. Three years later, the famous bubonic or "Black" plague swept northern Europe; and a decade later, diabetes first appeared.[13]

During the nineteenth century, as the consumption of refined flour and sugar grew still more widespread, the incidence of diabetes greatly increased, and the disease's typical progress through acidosis and coma became fairly well known; but the anatomical origin of the problem eluded researchers. (At different points in the early years of diabetes research, the disease was attributed to problems in the liver, stomach, blood, nervous system and kidneys.) Then in 1889, two Russian researchers, Minkowski and von Mering, made an epochal discovery quite by chance. To settle a dispute over the role of the pancreas, they removed a number of dogs' pancreases to see if they could live without them. Not only did the dogs die, but they all first developed the unmistakable symptoms of diabetes. Soon it was suggested that the Islets of Langerhans (discovered 20 years earlier) might secrete a hormone, dubbed "insulin" after the Latin for "islet," a lack of which might be causing the disease.

By this time the concept of hormone deficiencies was well established; and medical science had developed the therapeutic approach of using animal sources to supplement the deficient hormones, as a sort of chemical extension of the draft animal concept.[14] The race then began to produce a usable extract of the hypothetical insulin. At that time, according to E. M. Abrahamson, "Nearly every laboratory had at least one person making extracts of pancreases obtained from local abattoirs (slaughter-houses), experimental animals, and autopsy material, in order to obtain the elusive insulin. Everyone knew it was there, but no one was able to get a workable extract."[15] The problem was that the *exocrine* (non-hormone secreting) portion of the pancreas secretes protein-digesting enzymes; and insulin, being itself a protein, would be digested and destroyed by those same enzymes during the process of removing the organ. This is the reason that insulin-taking diabetics still need to inject their insulin. If taken orally, it would be completely digested before reaching the bloodstream.

The race was finally won in 1921 by two Canadians, Frederick Banting and his assistant Charles Best. They solved the digestive enzyme dilemma by tying off the pancreatic ducts that normally carry that digestive fluid to the intestine. Backing up, the fluid would destroy its own host organ, leaving the Islets of Langerhans intact. The remaining portion of the pancreas was then removed, and the insulin extracted.[16]

Banting and Best later received a Noble prize for their discovery; and 1921 was hailed as the beginning of a new era for diabetics. However, this new era was to contain some unpleasant surprises for the diabetic community.

The Insulin Era

By this time, medicine had begun to conquer infectious illness, and it was hoped that insulin would prove to be such a "magic bullet" for diabetes, which was fast growing from a fairly obscure disorder to a health problem of major proportions. Unfortunately, this soon proved to be an overly simplistic hope.

Prior to the insulin era, the diagnosis of diabetes amounted to a death sentence. Within weeks, or at the most years, after initial diagnosis, the patient inevitably succumbed to the horrible wasting, coma and death by ketoacidosis. The introduction of commercial insulin, and later in 1936 of long-term acting insulin, gave diabetics a reprieve; but oddly enough, the overall diabetic mortality rate hardly declined. The chart below, for example, shows the increase in diabetes-related deaths in England during the twenties and thirties: insulin was introduced between 1926 and 1928, yet there is no change whatsoever in the increasing mortality. This trend still continues today, over half a century later.

Year	Deaths per million
1920	110
1922	119
1925	112
1926	115
(insulin introduced)	
1928	131
1929	142
1931	145

Source: *Sugar Blues*, p. 83.

Researchers soon realized that although injections of swine or cattle insulin could provide the diabetic with enough *exogenous* (not self-produced) insulin to halt the process of deadly ketoacidosis, it didn't correct the underlying metabolic imbalance. Death was not avoided, only postponed —death not from coma, but from a range of complications that diabetes seemed to foster, such as heart attack, gangrene and even, in fairly rare instances, insulin shock from an overdose of the new drug.

For the diabetic, the insulin era has offered an "out of the frying pan and into the fire" dilemma. Routine injections of insulin save the patient from certain death by coma, yet have opened up an entirely new realm of health problems.[17] Banting's discovery of insulin set the stage for a renewed effort on the behalf of the scientific community to understand and treat this elusive disease.

What is Diabetes?

Strictly speaking, diabetes is not one disease but a full spectrum of blood glucose disorders ranging from *pre-diabetes* or *suspected diabetes*—slightly high BG levels or a sluggish insulin response, but often without any overt symptoms—to full-blown *overt* or *clinical* diabetes. (The earlier or milder forms are also called *latent, chronic* or *chemical* diabetes.)

The most common test for the detection and determination of diabetes is the "Oral Glucose Tolerance Test" (OGTT): the patient's blood is examined for glucose content after fasting for a period of hours, and again at regular intervals for several hours after consuming a "load" of pure glucose. The normal range for BG is from 80–120 mg percent. In the morning (after the night's fast) the BG is usually at the lower end of this scale. It tends to rise slightly after eating, and begins to level out again as soon as the pancreas begins to respond with insulin. A BG level that rises to over 130 mg percent after a glucose "load" is considered diabetic; diagnosis is usually made after two such occasions. A severe diabetic will have a BG level well over 130 mg percent even before taking the glucose (fasting BG level), and levels reaching even up to 1,000 mg percent are not too uncommon. Your ability to hold your glucose level within a normal range is called your "Glucose Tolerance." All diabetics suffer from a weakened glucose tolerance. (The OGTT, also called simply GTT, may be extended for four additional hours, usually when hypoglycemia is suspected.)

There are other common diabetes-related tests. Most diabetics regularly test their own urine for sugar to see whether their BG is "spilling over." This is done by passing chemically treated paper or sticks through the urine and examining them for color changes. These tests are unreliable, though, because urinary sugar may be present without diabetes, and in many diabetics, the BG may go dangerously high without registering in the urine. Tests for measuring the actual insulin content in the blood have also been developed, which are far more accurate.[18] Another recent advance is a method for measuring the amount of glucose attached to red blood cells, (*glycosylated hemoglobin*), which provides a far more meaningful profile of the past weeks' BG control, rather than the simple snapshot of the moment the GTT yields.

There are several types of diabetes within the fully developed (overt or clinical) category, which can be arranged on an ascending scale. There is often a confusion of terminology here; the list below follows the most commonly used terms, as revised by the NIH in 1979:

1. Impaired Glucose Tolerance (also called *Borderline* or *Sub-clinical* diabetes). Like latent diabetes, there are often no symptoms; but in this case, the GTT shows that the BG level is chronically at a definitely diabetic level. This is especially common in the elderly (in the Western hemisphere) and the obese. There is some debate as to whether or not this is likely to lead to more severe types of the disease. For one thing, this diagnosis is often made too late in life, or too soon before death from another disorder (such as heart disease), to follow the condition for long. One researcher has found that on the basis of the GTT, "We would reach the astonishing conclusion that the majority of elderly people have diabetes"[19]; another flatly states that this majority is "nearly 100 percent."[20]

2. *Gestational Diabetes.* Since the more yin hormones secreted during the second half of pregnancy tend to work against the pancreas, pregnancy often "unmasks" a hidden case of diabetes. When the mother has an abnormally high BG, the fetus often responds with an excess of insulin. Since insulin's anabolic action is largely responsible for the developing child's rapid growth, a history of giving birth to very large babies (over 9–10 pounds) is sometimes an indicator of borderline diabetes. This is another illustration of yin and yang. An overly expanded baby is a yin sign, indicating an excess of yin in the mother's diet during pregnancy: those same dietary excesses are the root cause of diabetes.

3. *Secondary and Induced Diabetes.* In fairly rare cases, diabetes can appear as the result of another, unrelated disease, such as pancreatitis, pancreatic cancer or liver disease. Far more commonly, diabetes can be "induced" by medications used to treat other conditions. This type of problem is called an *iatrogenic* ("doctor-caused") illness. The table below lists some of the medications and drugs that can raise the BG or even create diabetes; the most common examples are dilantin, certain diuretics, cortisone and other steroids, and oral contraceptives. All of these substances are extremely expansive (yin).

Birth control pills act by putting the hormonal system into a constantly "pseudo-pregnant" mode: and as we just learned, the hormonal balance of pregnancy can serve to unmask a case of latent or borderline diabetes. As one expert has put it, "the effect of oral contraceptives on carbohydrate metabolism is profound."[21] An often-cited study shows that "grossly diabetic" GTTs are observed in 15–40 percent of women taking oral contraceptives, and 80 percent showed a "lesser degree" of glucose intolerance. The birth control pill also creates an artificial resistance to the action of insulin; and four out of five women who are thus affected do not fully return to normal after stropping the pill.

The diabetogenic effect of steroids such as cortisone is easy to understand: all these medications are related to the more yin hormones which under normal circumstances keep the BG from going too low. In other words, they are naturally somewhat hyperglycemic; in fact, some of them have a temporarily neutralizing effect on hypoglycemia for this very reason. Adrenal glucocorticosteroids are often prescribed, for example, for patients with rheumatism or asthma.[22] However, if continued too long or dosed too high, they may easily cause induced diabetes.

BG-Affecting Drugs and Medications[23]

Increase BG	Lower BG
(potentially diabetes inducing)	(potentially hypoglycemia inducing)
dilantin	aspirin
thyazide diuretics	barbituates
chlorpromazine	bishydroxycoumarin
epinephrine (adrenaline)	chloramphenicol
indomethocin	MAO inhibitors
adrenal steroids (cortisone,	oxyphenbutazone
cortisol, etc.)	PAS & INH
androgens	phenylbutazone
estrogens	phenyramidol
oral contraceptives	probenecid
growth hormone	propranolol HCL
thyroxin	sodium salicylate
glucagon	biguanidines*
ACTH	sulfonyureas*
LSD	
marijuana	
niacin (Vitamin B$_3$)	
ascorbic acid (Vitamin C)	

* These two classes of drugs are often used as oral hypoglycemics in the treatment of Type II diabetes.

Primary Diabetes

The last two categories of overt diabetes are by far the most common types, and are considered together as constituting *Primary Diabetes*.

Type I diabetes, affecting about 10 percent of the diabetic population, is diabetes at its most deadly. Often explosively sudden, it usually appears in childhood and may run a rapid course to ketoacidosis and death if not quickly caught and treated. Once Type I diabetes is diagnosed the patient almost always requires daily injections of insulin for the rest of his life.

A sudden loss of weight or appeitite, unusually great thirst or urination, bedwetting, and an unusual tendency towards fatigue, lethargy or crankiness are the most common early clues. A full list of "early warning signs," widely circulated by the Juvenile Diabetes Foundation and other groups, is given in following table. However, these would more aptly be called "late" warning signs: it would of course be far preferable to detect a possible tendency towards diabetes years before it appears in acute form, and take steps towards prevention. It may be more easily corrected if detected during this "incubation"—but once fully developed, it is extremely difficult to reverse.

Diabetes: Warning Signs and Early Symptoms

Type I	*Type II*
frequent urination	frequent or nocturnal urination
abnormal thirst & hunger	obesity
sudden weight loss	drowsiness (easily fatigued)
sudden irritability	blurred vision
weakness & fatigue	tingling or numbness in
nausea & vomiting	hands & feet
abdominal pain	itching & skin infections
shortness of breath	slow healing of cuts (esp. feet)
	Pruritis Vulvae (vaginal infection)
	history of abnormally large babies
	amenorrhea (cessation of periods)
	cramps in calves, legs
	poor memory, weak thinking

The onset of Type I is often somewhat less sudden among teenagers and young adults; it is also quite rare in the very young of Japan and tropical countries.[24] Type I is also referred to as *Juvenile-onset, insulin-dependent* and *ketoacidosis-prone* diabetes.

Type II diabetes (also called *mature-onset, non-insulin-dependent* and *ketoacidosis-resistant*) is the most prevalent form, affecting up to 90 percent of the diabetic population. Usually developing after the age of forty (though like Type I, it can appear at any age), Type II does not usually require routine insulin injections. Unlike Type I patients, most Type II diabetics do secrete their own insulin—in fact, they usually secrete more than a non-diabetic! The insulin they secrete, though, isn't as effective as it should be, and though they are not prone to the severe problem of ketoacidosis, they suffer nonetheless from a chronically high BG level and its associated complications.

The distinction between these two types is one of the great diabetes puzzles—because of the differences in their pattern of development and in the state of the pancreas and its hormones, the two types are often considered as two entirely different diseases, with different causes. Yet, if these two are in fact different, how can we account for the fact that they ultimately run the same course of symptoms and complications?

In reality, these anatomical differences are more superficial concerns and do not reflect truly different causes. The underlying cause of both types is the same, namely an excessive consumption of overly yin food and drink. The differences between the two, as we shall see presently, stem largely from how much of those items are consumed and at what point in the person's life.

Most Type II diabetics are overweight (obesity is considered one of the major contributing factors), and simply losing weight can often temper the severity and speed of the disease and its symptoms. In addition to diet, oral hypoglycemics (BG-lowering medications) are commonly used to keep the BG within tolerable limits. Like insulin therapy, though, these medications do not cure the disease.

Oral Drugs

There are two schools of thought regarding the proper treatment for Type II diabetes. Some physicians feel that patients should do their utmost to maintain as normal a BG level as possible through diet and weight control, while others argue that this is too much to expect of the patient, and that oral drugs are a more practical solution.

There are two types of oral hypoglycemics: *sulfonyureas*, including tolbutamide (marketed under the name Orinase), tolazamide (Tolinase), acetohexamide (Dymelor) and chlorpropramide (Diabinase); and *biguanidines*, including Phenformin and Metformin. The blood glucose lowering properties of the sulfa drugs, discovered quite by accident in 1942, seem to work through their direct action on the beta cells of the pancreas. The biguanidines do not affect the pancreas, but rather work by reducing absorption of carbohydrates in the intestine and inhibiting the functions of the kidneys, adrenals and liver.

When the first commercial hypoglycemic agent tolbutamide (Orinase) was introduced in 1956, it was found effective in 80–85 percent of the patients treated; the other 15–20 percent experienced unexplained failure.

After one month of use, it was found to stop working in 25 percent of the patients, and after several years of use, 90 percent failed to experience continued results.[25] The reason for this dropping off of effectiveness may be that the beta cells, which are usually already overworked in Type II diabetics, are eventually exhausted by the drug's added stimulation. The known side-effects of the sulfa hypoglycemics can include: diarrhea, headache, heartburn, loss of appetite, nausea, vomiting, stomach upset, liver or blood problems, worsening of pre-existing problems with the kidneys, liver or thyroid, infection, seizure, swelling, water retention and general weakness.

The hypoglycemic effect of Phenformin was first discovered in 1918. However, early attempts to use the drug in treating diabetes resulted in cases of severe kidney and liver damage, and the drug was hastily dropped. With the introduction of the sulfa group in the 1950's interest was rekindled, and new, less toxic versions of biguanidines were soon on the market. Though not as severe as the catastrophic impact of the earlier drug, the new biguanidines are not without their problems. Two-third of patients using Phenformin develop "gastrointestinal intolerance," which may include nausea, loss of appetite, a metallic taste in the mouth, and bouts of diarrhea or vomiting.[26]

The major problem with the oral drugs has been the considerable doubt as to whether they do actually reduce the risk of diabetic complications. To answer that question and resolve the debate over the drugs' use, a major study was launched in 1961, the University Study Diabetes Project (UGDP). One of the first large-scale trials of its kind, the UGDP's seven-year study followed over 800 Type II diabetics undergoing different therapies.[27] The study's findings, that the oral drugs tested were generally ineffective and if anything may have actually increased the risk of heart attack, touched off a raging debate which has still not been resolved.[28]

The Complications of Diabetes

Far more deadly than diabetes itself are the various secondary problems that often accompany the illness. These include the following:

1. *Cardiovascular Disease.* Normally, insulin serves to remove both glucose and circulating fats from the bloodstream. In the diabetic, of course, that doesn't happen, and the whole circulatory system usually bears the burden of this abuse. Diabetics are twice as likely as non-diabetics to die from this class of illness (already the Number One killer in society at large); and 50 percent of all American heart attacks are due to diabetes. In addition to the generally common problems of heart

attack, stroke and sclerosis of the large vessels ("hardening of the arteries"), diabetics suffer from a unique problem: *microangiopathy*. Literally "disease of the tiny vessels," microangiopathy is a degeneration of the fine network of blood vessels permeating the body's more yin sensitive tissues. This results in a thickening of delicate membranes and an increasing porousness and weakness of the vessels, which ultimately leads to a total breakdown of the tissue, especially appearing in the kidneys, eyes, nerves and periphery (skin and limbs).

2. *Kidney Problems.* The kidneys are responsible for "dumping" excess blood sugar, and are among the first organs to suffer the long-term effects of microangiopathy. Diabetics are seventeen times more likely to have kidney failure, which kills 40 percent of all Type I patients. The problem is compounded by the fact that common kidney treatments (dialysis, transplant and diuretics) are all made difficult or impossible by the diabetes itself.

3. *Eye Disorders.* The leading cause of new blindness, diabetes causes 5,000 new cases per year and makes Type I patients twenty-five times more likely than the general population to go blind. Common complications include *glaucoma*, a building up of water pressure in the eye with a progressive hardening of the eyeball; *cataracts*, concentrated areas of opaque fatty build-up on the eye's surface; and *diabetic retinitis* or inflammation of the retina. By far the worst problem is *retinopathy*, the degeneration of the retina or optic nerve itself.

4. *Neuropathy.* The brain and all nervous tissue are especially sensitive to glucose. A high BG gradually impairs the functioning of not only the optic and renal (kidney) nerves, but also of the sensory and motor nerves leading to the limbs. For many diabetics this effect is first felt as a trembling or partial loss of sensation in the legs or hands; after ten years, nine out of ten patients experience some degree of nerve deadening in the lower legs. This may be preceded by a period of excruciating pain, especially at night. Sometimes even the pressure of bedsheets touching the legs brings on intolerable agony. Diabetic neuropathy may also affect the autonomic nervous system, which controls many of the body's unconscious functions, leading to a decrease in perspiration, impotence and digestive difficulties. It can also affect the brain itself, causing a loss of will power, chronic depression, and other personality or behavioral changes.

5. *Susceptibility to Infection.* The blood's overly rich sugar concentration lends itself to infection, which can be very difficult to control. Dia-

betics are repeatedly warned, for example, to protect their feet with great care, and with good reason; uncontrollable infection leading to gangrene is five times more common in diabetics—and of the feet, seventy times more common! Diabetic gangrene, in fact, is the most common reason for amputation, which is forty times more likely for diabetics than for non-diabetics. Other types of infection, including skin abscesses, meningitis and ear infections, are also prevalent in diabetics; vaginal yeast infections and recurrent skin problems are often the first presenting symptoms of diabetes.

6. *Digestive Disorders.* Diarrhea, nausea, anorexia, appendicitis, megacolon (expanded large intestine), and other problems of the stomach, small intestine and large intestine are all more common in diabetics.

7. *Problems with Pregnancy and Childbearing.* Before the days of insulin injections, diabetic women rarely lived to childbearing age. In the twentieth century, pregnancy has been found to pose special problems for diabetic mothers. For example, the incidence of stillbirth, birth defects (spina bifida, clubfoot, missing digits and others) and glucose problems in the child are far higher among diabetics. The situation has drastically improved in the past 15 years; only a decade ago, the rate of perinatal mortality (death during or shortly before or after birth) stood at 15–20 percent—today it is down to about 5 percent. Still, diabetic mothers are rarely allowed to go to full term (with the exception of Gestational Diabetes): the risks of complications, for the mother or the child, are considered too great.

8. *Sexual Problems.* Diabetes is often associated with impotence, due to an impairment of the autonomic nerve and sexual hormone balance. The entire genito-urinary tract is also more susceptible to infection.

9. *Insulin-related Problems.* Finally, there are a number of difficulties brought on by the treatment itself. The most dangerous is *insulin shock*, a profound state of low BG (hypoglycemia) brought on by an accidental overdose of insulin. (A sudden change in the body's need for insulin, such as occurs after unusually strenuous exercise, may also render the normal dosage an overdose in effect.) A small percentage of diabetics die from insulin overdose. One of the problems is that insulin shock, unlike the diabetic coma of ketoacidosis, comes on very rapidly and it is easily mistaken for diabetic coma or, more commonly, for a case of drunkenness or drug abuse. Diabetics usually wear a bracelet stating that if found unconscious, the person should be given some-

thing with sugar in it to revive him. Because the onset of insulin shock is so sudden, it is essential that the diabetic learn to recognize the feeling right away, in time to take action before he is rendered unconscious. Insulin therapy may also create local problems at the site of injection, such as an accumulation of fat or a withering of the skin. Some patients also develop an allergy to the insulin itself, though this is rare.

Perhaps the most profound problem with insulin treatment, though, is that the patient becomes an addict out of necessity. Unlike the person addicted to alcohol, drugs or other substances, however, there is no way to "dry out" or "take the cure": it is an addiction for life. The discovery of insulin was certainly a blessing; yet it is a mixed blessing. Often regarded as a "cure" of sorts, it actually allows the underlying disorder to continue its devastating course. Seen in a larger context, insulin contains the hidden danger of any treatment that controls symptoms without addressing the original cause: it may soften our sense of urgency and tend to undermine our efforts to find and correct that cause.

Current Medical Views on the Cause of Diabetes ———

Finding the cause of diabetes has proved to be one of the great medical riddles of the twentieth century. A tremendous amount of time, effort and expense has been poured into the problem since the beginning of the insulin era. "In almost no other field of medicine has there been so much investigative research along so many different lines in the past few years," wrote one researcher in 1980.[29] Yet there are still no clear, generally agreed upon conclusions as to the disease's cause, or even as to exactly what happens in the body to trigger its complications.

The classical explanation for diabetes is that some people have an inherited weakness in the pancreas; and in those with a genetic predisposition, an infection (or possible a series of infections) somehow causes irreversible damage to the islet cells. Regional "outbreaks" of diabetes appearing after small-scale epidemics of mumps or other viral infections have seemed to support this idea.[30]

More recent research has suggested a third factor: diabetics may manufacture antibodies which attack the pancreas instead of fighting off infection. These pancreas-directed antibodies seem to appear in the diabetic's blood long before the disease actually develops, gradually lowering the patient's insulin output, until some factor (again, possibly a virus) finally triggers the full-blown condition.

However, there are major problems with this view. For one thing, only about 5 percent of the children born to diabetic couples develop the disease (if only one parent has diabetes, the chances are even slimmer), and two-third of all diabetics have no family history of diabetes whatsoever. In fact, the risk of genetic factors may be virtually zero; or, as one authority puts it, "maybe we are all genetic diabetics."[31] If genetics is not a major factor, then why would an infection trigger such devastating destruction in some people and not in others? The same problem appears with the antibody or *auto-immune* theory: if pancreas-directed antibodies cause the disease's progress, why do some have them and others not? Attempts to use immune-suppressing drugs to combat the antibodies have so far not produced encouraging results; and such treatments raise a number of ethical and scientific issues: the drugs themselves can produce serious side-effects, including diabetes itself![32]

The classical model was dealt a major blow in the 1950's with the development of a new method for testing the blood's actual insulin content. Up to that time it was assumed that all diabetics suffered from a lack of insulin—now it was found that the vast majority of Type II diabetics do secrete their own insulin, and in fact, secrete far more than normal. This discovery has led to a major reexamination of all the possible factors involved in glucose metabolism—from the pancreas itself and its hormones, to the body cell's reception of insulin, to possible imbalances in other endocrine functions—to try and pinpoint the cause. The two most common lines of thought are described below:

An Imbalance of Insulin Antagonists. Since there are so many hormones that naturally work to counter insulin, the idea that excessive insulin antagonists may be a key factor in diabetes has received a lot of attention. Glucagon, the pancreas' other major hormone, was discovered two years after insulin, but has only in the past few years emerged as a major focus of study: most diabetics have been found to have high levels of the hormone in their blood. (The normal function of glucagon, remember, is to raise the BG when it is too low, and glucagon is often injected for emergency treatment of insulin shock.) Because of the high diabetes rates in patients with hypersecretion of pituitary growth hormone (gigantism and acromegaly) and thyroid hormone (goiter), these two hormones are among the many other substances suspected to be involved. These two are both more yin hormones.

Defects in Insulin Use. The other common line of thinking is that the body's cells may be unable to use insulin effectively, probably due to obesity. For insulin to introduce sugar, fat or protein molecules into a cell it needs to fasten to a tiny molecule called an *insulin receptor*; these receptors are located on the outer and inner membranes of body cells. It appears, though, that the cell itself can alter the number of its receptors. In fat cells, this number goes down as the cell increases in size, while in a muscle cell, it goes up as the cell grows. Obesity (particularly coupled with lack of exercise) results in an overall decrease in the number of receptor sites, which amounts to "insulin resistance"—though the Type II patient secretes the hormone, his cells can't accept it.

Other Theories. Another molecule has been discovered that helps introduce insulin to its receptors. Called the *Glucose Tolerance Factor* (GTF), it is composed of three *niacins* (Vitamin B_3) and two *glutamic acids* (one of the constituents of protein) connected by a chromium atom. Primary grown yeast, which contains GTF, has been administered to diabetics and caused the appearance of insulin shock, suggesting that a chronic deficiency in GTF or dietary chromium may be another key factor.

Other research has suggested that the insulin itself may determine the receptor's "affinity" (ability to accept insulin). This suggests that in diabetics who do produce insulin, perhaps a weakness or defective quality of that insulin prevents its proper use. Again, other researchers claim that there is a defect in the body cells themselves, and not the insulin or its receptors, that is at fault. For example, an excess of triglycerides in the blood can cause the fat molecules to lodge on the outer walls of blood and other cells, blocking off the receptor sites. A high level of blood triglycerides, in turn, can be caused by the consumption of excessive fats or *fructose*, a simple sugar found in fruit, honey and *sucrose* (table sugar).

The Macrobiotic View of the Cause of Diabetes———

As we have already seen, it is an overly yin diet that weakens the pancreas and other functions, leading to the problem of diabetes. Another important factor influencing the distinction between the different types of the illness is the particular nature of the person's constitution. Already largely determined by the time of birth, one's *constitution* consists of those relatively permanent physical characteristics influenced by the quality of the parents' reproductive cells and of the mother's diet during pregnancy. Since the strengths and qualities of our reproductive cells are constantly affected by the quality of our blood, which in turn is determined largely by our daily diet, the characteristics we pass on to our offspring are profoundly affected by our way of eating prior to conception. In fact, many of the characteristics usually attributed to heredity may actually be determined more by a certain pattern of diet passed down through one's family, and may be changed in only one generation by a significant departure from the family's general way of eating.

A more yang constitution is characterized by such features as a sturdier frame with thicker, more heavy-set bones, a more square, broad face, broader shoulders and a stockier appearance, smaller facial features grouped closely together, more square palms with shorter, thicker fingers, and a shorter stature. Signs of a more yin constitution include a more slender, delicate bone structure with more elongated features, a taller height, a thinner, more vertically oriented face, sloping shoulders and a more slight appearance, larger eyes and mouth or a longer nose, with the facial features spread more widely apart, and more narrow, long palms with thin, long fingers.[33]

Type II (Obese). An obese Type II diabetic (the majority) is generally an individual with a somewhat more yang constitution, and may suffer from more yang conditional problems earlier in life, such as heart disorders caused by the overconsumption of eggs, meat and salted foods. It is only later in life that he begins to consume inordinate amounts of more yin extremes, or to take diabetogenic drugs in the treatment of other problems. The resulting more yin condition creates a greater demand for insulin; however, the progressive weakening of the pancreas begins to undermine the normal process of transforming proinsulin into insulin. The result is a greater quantity but weaker, more yin and less effective quality of insulin.[34] After eliminating the offending dietary items and adopting a macrobiotic way of eating, this type of diabetes is usually reversed fairly easily in a short period of time.

Type I (Juvenile). Unlike Type II, Type I diabetes is strongly influenced by extremely yin factors in the parents' diet just prior to conception and in the mother's diet during pregnancy. This is best illustrated by the following study:

> Researchers in Iceland recently noted an odd fact: diabetic boys in Iceland often have birthdays in October. Sensing this was more than coincidence, one doctor studied the problem and arrived at a startling conclusion. The winter holiday celebrations in Iceland usually include feasting on a particular type of smoked mutton—a dish which nowadays contains several nitrosamines, extremely yin substances closely related to a compound (streptozotocin) commonly used in laboratory experiments to induce diabetes for research purposes. An October birthday suggests a January conception: just after the winter holidays. When the researcher fed the same mutton to adult mice just prior to mating, every sixth male offspring developed diabetes.[35]

Nitrosamines, of course, are only one example of extreme yin. A wide variety of very expansive foods, consumed by the parents prior to conception or by the mother during pregnancy, can create the tendency towards diabetes in the offspring. This yin constitutional factor. however, only produces that tendency. It is the overconsumption of very yin food and drink in the child's own diet that usually causes this inborn weakness to actually develop into diabetes. These items especially include: milk and dairy products, sugary pastries and candies, chocolate, soft drinks, ice cream, honey, tropical fruits and their juices, and refined flour products (white bread, "cold cereals" and baked goods.) Even with such an inborn tendency, a person need not develop diabetes if he or she follows a balanced, moderate diet and completely avoids those foods.

When Type I diabetes has already recently developed, it is often still possible to reverse the course of the illness through proper eating. However, the longer the disease is present, the harder it becomes to achieve a complete recovery. Still, even a long time Type I patient can usually reduce insulin requirements to a fraction of their previous level, and avoid the possibility of diabetic complications, by adopting a macrobiotic approach under proper guidance.

Type II (Non-obese) and Type I (Adult). These two types fall in between the older, obese Type II and infant or juvenile-onset Type I; moreover, the borderline between non-obese Type II and the upper age bracket of Type I is somewhat vague. In this category, the person usually has a generally more yin constitution (but without the extremely yin constitutional factor present in younger Type I patients), and therefore succumbs to the effects of a more yin diet earlier in life than the more constitutionally yang obese patient; and it may take much longer to recover normal health after beginning to follow a macrobiotic approach than for the obese Type II patient.

Three Types of Diabetes and Corresponding Constitutional Factors

Type:	Type I	Type I (adult) and Type II (non-obese)	Type II (obese)
Degree:	most yin	less yin	least yin
Average age of onset:	infancy—teens	young—mid adult	middle—old age
Constitutional factor:	extreme yin taken by parents just prior to or just after conception	generally more yin constitution	generally more yang constitution

Yin and Yang and Diabetic Complications ———————

The extremely yin condition of diabetes affects not only the pancreas but also the other glands, organs, the blood and the body as a whole. Consequently, the degeneration of diabetes tends to spread to more yin regions— the periphery, including the skin, limbs and peripheral vessels and nerves. (The opposite is true in hypoglycemia, where symptoms tend to gather in a more inward direction.) For example, the microangiopathy so unique to diabetics is a degeneration of the most yin, differentiated vessels, while the non-diabetic (more yang) vascular disease patient is affected in the more yang central arteries. To understand why the brain, nerve and eye cells are also particularly affected, we need to understand the way insulin normally works in terms of yin and yang.

Fig. 12.   Cellular glucose metabolism: normal (A–C) and diabetic (D–E).

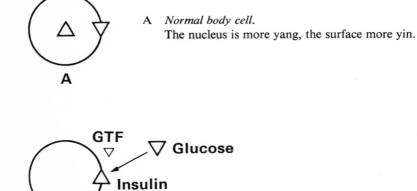

A   *Normal body cell.*
    The nucleus is more yang, the surface more yin.

B. *Normal cell metabolism.* The introduction of insulin (yang) allows the cell surface (normally yin) to attract yin glucose. Insulin receptors (yang) and GTF (yin) also play roles in this process.

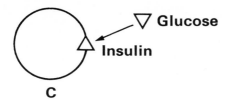

C

C. *Normal brain, nerve and eye cell metabolism.* Brain, nerve and eye cells, all more yang, can normally attract glucose even without the yang catalyst of insulin.

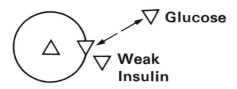

D. *In diabetes,* insulin is either weak (yin) or absent. The yin cell surface and yin glucose repel each other, and glucose moves out to peripheral circulation, causing complications.

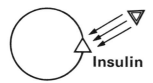

E. *In diabetes,* the yang brain, nerve and eye cells consume excessive amounts of glucose, causing complications.

Glucose is yin, and to enter a body cell it must first come into contact with and penetrate the cell's outer wall, its most yin, peripheral part. Since similar energies normally repel one another, a yang catalyst is needed. Insulin fills this need, attaching to the cell wall and attracting the yin glucose. Glucose Tolerance Factor (GTF) and the insulin receptors, which are respectively more yin and more yang, also play roles in this process.

The cells of the brain, nerve and eye, however, are particularly yang cells; in fact, it is their yang nature that serves the function of attracting the more yin, short wave energies of light, thought and neural impulse. Because they are more yang than other body cells, they do not normally require insulin in order to accept and metabolize glucose.

In the case of diabetes, insulin becomes more yin or disappears altogether, so the blood's glucose is repelled by the cells' surface and remains in the bloodstream, then expanding out to the body's peripheral circulation and causing the above cited complications.

However, the absence or weakness of insulin doesn't interfere with the glucose metabolism of the brain, eye and nerve cells. Quite the contrary, they thirstily drink in the overabundance of blood glucose. Like a person made very yang by spending several days in the hot desert and then greedily drinking his fill of cold water, this overconsumption by the more yang cells easily causes them to become extremely yin and weak. When this process repeats itself over time, it naturally leads to degeneration of these cells as well.

[1] Brothers, p. 19.
[2] Brothers, p. 33 and Bloom, p. 16.
[3] Charles Nechemias, M.D., in his introduction to *The Sugar Disease: Diabetes*, Silverstein.
[4] R. H. Major, ed., *Classic Descriptions of Disease*, Springfield, Ill., Thomas, 1932, p. 186.
[5] Trowell, p. 23.
[6] G. D. Campbell, *Nutrition and Disease*, 1973. Part III, Appendix to the Hearings of the United States Senate, Series 73/ND3. Quoted in Dufty, p. 78.
[7] Vasopressin is a more yang hormone secreted by the anterior pituitary.
[8] *East West Journal*, p. 26.
[9] Trowell, p. 24.
[10] Trowell, p. 24.
[11] Trowell, p. 14.
[12] *Pharmaceutice Rationalis*, 1674, Sir Thomas Willis.
[13] Dufty, p. 74. For a detailed account of the appearance and growing role of refined sugar in modern health and economic life, please see Dufty's *Sugar Blues*, pp. 26–94.
[14] For example, a condition called "myxedema" or Gull's disease, in which a subnormal secretion of thyroxin from the thyroid causes lethargy, obesity, a coarsening of features and other conditions, had been successfully treated with extracts of thyroid from sheep and cattle.
[15] Abrahamson, p. 17.
[16] This process, though it did succeed in isolating insulin, produces far too little hormone for commercial use. Another process was soon developed to treat the pancreas

with dilute hydrochloric acid, inactivating the enzyme (trypsin), before extracting the insulin. (Abrahamson, p. 20.) Today, the glands are frozen immediately after surgery, which inactivates the trypsin, and shipped to their processing plants.

[17] This is emerging as a common theme in modern treatments of degenerative disorders: some chemotherapeutic treatments are often more deadly than the cancers they are used to relieve.

[18] For example, insulin is made in the pancreas by splitting apart a peptide (protein) chain called "proinsulin," consisting of an A-peptide and B-peptide connected by a C-peptide. When insulin is formed, the C-peptide chains are discarded into the blood; testing the blood for its level of C-peptides shows whether and how much insulin is being produced.

[19] Bloom, p. 16.

[20] Brothers, p. 33.

[21] Brothers, p. 67.

[22] These conditions, not surprisingly, are often associated with hypoglycemia.

[23] Compiled from Light, p. 14, *Runner's World*, Jan. 1984, p. 70, and others.

[24] Trowell, p. 25.

[25] Bloom, p. 36 ff.

[26] Bloom, p. 36 ff.

[27] Out of five groups, one took insulin, three took different drugs, and one took placebos.

[28] *Science*, March 16, 1979.

[29] Dr. Charles Nechemias, in his introduction to *Silver*, p. 10.

[30] The virus-plus-inherited-tendency model has been suggested for a number of other major diseases such as cancer.

[31] Brothers, p. 50.

[32] *Science News*, February 19, 1983.

[33] For a complete discussion of constitutional types and the factors that determine them, please refer to *How to See Your Health* by the author.

[34] This problem of quality versus quantity occurs in many other contexts. For example, the use of extensive hybridizing and petro-chemical fertilizers of the "Green Revolution" in modern agriculture has créated food crops with a greater volume of yield, but a much weaker nutritional quality and resistance to environmental factors.

[35] *American Health*, May/June 1983, p. 35.

3. Hypoglycemia ▬▬▬▬▬▬▬▬▬▬▬▬

In 1924, only three years after Banting and Best had successfully produced insulin for use in the treatment of diabetes, a doctor at the University of Alabama began to notice a recurring pattern of hunger, weakness, anxiety and heart palpitations in some of this patients. By now familiar with the new insulin therapy, Dr. Seale Harris recognized that these were the typical symptoms of insulin shock which accompany the rapid fall in blood sugar caused by an accidental overdose of insulin. However, none of these particular patients were taking insulin, in fact, they were not even diabetic! Dr. Harris concluded that this must be a disorder caused by the *hypersecretion* of insulin, and called the new "disease" *hyperinsulinism*; later that year he published his findings in the Journal of the American Medical Association.

We have since learned that hypoglycemia is not necessarily caused by an excess of insulin, just as diabetes is not usually caused by an simple lack of insulin. Hypoglycemia is actually not a disease, but a "syndrome," a condition that can arise from a number of different origins, including an excess of insulin, a deficiency of insulin antagonists, or other, non-hormonal mechanisms. Whatever the cause, the result is the same: the blood doesn't contain enough circulating glucose to properly nourish the body's cells.

A diagnosis of hypoglycemia is usually made by extending the standard 2-hour GTT to 4, 5 or 6 hours, as it often takes several hours after eating for the BG to drop to its lowest point. But there is still some debate over at what point "normal" ends and hypoglycemia begins. Cahill's Encyclopedia of Medicine defines hypoglycemia as "a blood glucose level of 40 mg percent or lower, so that the central nervous system is impaired."[1] This refers, though, only to the most severe (and fortunately, most rare) types of hypoglycemia; the symptoms of hypoglycemia can also occur when the BG falls below 60–80 mg percent. The range from 70 mg percent down to 40 mg percent has been called a "margin of safety,"[2] where the body begins to respond in an emergency mode, but is not yet in acute or immediate danger. It is this type of more subtle hypoglycemia that is so prevalent.

A commonly held view is that it is not the exact level but the speed with which the level drops, or how far it drops, that determines the body's reaction and creates hypoglycemia.[3] Further, what is a normal level for one person may not be normal for another: dropping to a level of 90 mg percent (which is well within the "normal" range) may cause hypoglycemic symptoms in a person whose BG is normally 95 mg percent or higher. Also, it is not unusual for someone with transient or sporadic hypoglycemia to show a completely normal GTT during a visit to the doctor's office.[4] These common views may be summarized as follows:

1. A BG of below 40 mg percent unquestionably indicates severe, sometimes even life-threatening hypoglycemia.
2. A BG of from 80 mg percent down to 40 mg percent indicates a hypoglycemic condition which may be of different levels of severity, sometimes clinically obvious and sometimes more subtle.
3. A BG in any range that shows unusually steep or rapid drops, or an uncharacteristically low reading of even several points, may indicate hypoglycemia of varying degrees of subtlety.
4. A person exhibiting several of the common symptoms of hypo-glycemia (which will be discussed shortly) but whose GTT reads normal may in fact suffer from the disorder.

What Happens in Hypoglycemia?

Hypoglycemia is often misleadingly called "low blood sugar"; conse-quently, with the resulting reasoning that eating more sugar will alleviate the condition, hypoglycemics are often told to carry sugar cubes or candy bars with them at all times (something like the inverse of the diabetic's ubiquitous insulin kit!)[1]. This type of logic points out a very serious mis-understanding of the nature of the disorder: the problem is not that the person doesn't eat enough glucose-containing foods, but that the body doesn't properly use the sugars it gets. In fact, many hypoglycemics eat plenty of carbohydrates of one form or another, but the metabolism is unbalanced so that the action of insulin is normally or overly strong, and the actions that oppose insulin are weakened.

What happens, then, to the glucose you absorb from the food you eat? Some of it is quickly burned as fuel, and the rest is vigorously stored away as glycogen or fat. While the diabetic's blood glucose accumulates until it reaches destructive levels, the hypoglycemic's overly yang system would soaks up glucose like a dry sponge. Normally, dropping glucose levels stimulate the adrenals to start pumping cortical hormones to the liver to retrieve glycogen and, if necessary, manufacture new fuels. In hypoglycemia, however, the blood-glucose raising mechanisms are often stagnated and don't operate smoothly. Unable to bring the level back up to normal, the natural response is an urge to take in new sources of glucose; a constant or frequent gnawing hunger is often the first noticeable symptom of hypoglycemia.

Unfortunately, though the next meal may bring the BG levels temporarily back up, this only triggers the overactive Islets to secrete still more insulin, leading again to a lowered BG level. This sequence can develop into a vicious cycle of wider and wider swings of raising and dropping glucose levels, requiring stronger and stronger stimulation to bring the levels up, with progressively more profound symptoms as they drop again.

The Symptoms of Hypoglycemia

For some people, hypoglycemia is an occasional problem triggered by an unusual stress, lack of sleep, unusually long period without eating (particularly if the person is using coffee, alcohol or a drug to fend off hunger and keep himself awake), or other unusually demanding circumstances. In others, it is a chronic condition that builds almost imperceptibly into a general background of poor health. The severity of the symptoms that usually accompany the condition depend on the severity and speed of the drop in blood glucose. A rapid drop, particularly to very low levels, prompts the powerful *adrenal medulla* (central portion) to secrete its "emergency hormone," adrenaline, into the blood, causing:

> rapid heartbeat (*tachycardia*) and accelerated breathing, clammy skin and sweating or chills, intense anxiety, fear or tension, and hunger or, in some cases, nausea.

These are the classic symptoms of insulin shock.[5]

Far more common are cases where the BG level drops too gradually to stimulate the emergency mechanism of adrenaline. In this case, the body is put on a "partial alert": the *adrenal cortex* (outer portion) secretes cortical hormones, which cause milder reactions:

> headache, confusion or disorientation, double or blurred vision, insatiable hunger, uncontrollable yawning, nervousness or lack of concentration, fatigue; (in rare cases, convulsion or coma).

If this condition persists and becomes a chronic response, it can generate further long-term symptoms, such as

> extreme pessimism, depression or a sense of futility and personal worthlessness, personality changes, restlessness and emotional instability, chronic fatigue, outbursts of temper or violence, susceptibility to colds, infection (especially persistent, low-grade infections) and a host of other, seemingly non-related mental and physical disorders.

The literature on hypoglycemia is replete with pages of lists of conditions commonly associated with low blood glucose. To cite just one of these sources, Marilyn Light, president of the Hypoglycemia Foundation in New York, lists the following problems as known "complications" associated with hypoglycemia:

addictions, alcoholism, allergies, arthritis, anxiety, convulsions, depression, high I.Q. children labeled as underachievers, incoordination, insomnia, juvenile delinquency, migraine headaches, frequent nightmares, suicidal tendencies, staggering, ulcerlike pains, weakness and light-headedness with or without fainting, fatigue and exhaustion, premenstrual tension syndrome (PMS).[6]

Organic Versus Functional Hypoglycemia

How common a role hypoglycemia may actually play in many of these disorders is an issue of some debate; in fact, some doctors hotly contest the idea that hypoglycemia is a common condition at all. This debate is often confused by the fact that there are two distinct versions of the condition: those that are caused by a clearly diagnosable, anatomical defect, and those that are not. The first class, termed "organic," is quite rare, and is quite well recognized by conventional medicine; the second may be referred to as *reactive, relative* or *functional* hypoglycemia. Organic hypoglycemia may be caused by a variety of diseases:

1. *Pancreatic Disease.* There are three types of pancreas disorder that can cause genuine hypoinsulinism. The rarest and most lethal is *insuloma*, a malignancy of the islet cells which frequently spreads throught the body causing an uncontrollable secretion of excess insulin. Benign tumors of the islets can also cause hypersecretion of insulin, as can a generalized enlargement of the tail of the pancreas, which is usually treated by removing a portion of the tail.

2. *Diseases of the Insulin Antagonists' Organs.* When any of the organs or glands that secrete insulin antagonists are impaired by disease, normal levels of insulin may become over-effective. Common examples are liver cirrhosis, hepatitis or obstructive jaundice; adrenal cortex insufficiency of "Addison's disease"; hypothyroidism (myxedema or "Gull's disease"); and disease of the pituitary (dwarfism, pituitary cachexia or "Simmond's disease"). For therapy, an extract of the underactive gland is often administered, though in many cases this doesn't provide complete or permanent relief.

3. *Cancer.* Cancer tends to absorb large amounts of the blood's glucose for its own metabolism, and can thereby starve the host metabolism, leading to low blood glucose and general wasting.

4. *Children's Hypoglycemia.* "Glycogen storage disease" is a rare disorder of the young, in which the child lacks the enzymes needed to convert glycogen into glucose. Some children are also highly sensitive to the simple sugars fructose (present in large amounts in fruits, honey and table sugar) and *galactose* (present in large quantities in milk), and develop hypoglycemia as a result. Both these problems tend to recede with normal ageing.[7]

Reactive and Functional Hypoglycemia

In organic hypoglycemia, the BG is constantly depressed; this is also called *fasting* hypoglycemia. Reactive means that the person's metabolism overreacts to the blood glucose raising stimulus of eating. There are three commonly known versions of this syndrome: post-operative hypoglycemia occurs when the digestive system is surgically bypassed so that food empties directly from the esophagus into the small intestine; the rapid absorption of glucose causes the pancreas to overreact.

Reactive hypoglycemia can also be caused by the progressively weakening islet cells of pre-diabetes: an initially sluggish insulin response to glucose from a meal causes mild hyperglycemia at first, followed by an overreaction within several hours which brings the blood glucose down below normal levels. (Some physicians believe that this condition precedes virtually every case of fully developed overt diabetes.)

Finally, there is the chronic condition known as functional hypoglycemia. By far the most common variety, this is what is usually meant when people speak of hypoglycemia. Medically speaking, there is no known cause; one doctor stated in 1968 that ". . . until recently many physicians were not sure that there was such a disease . . . [it has] not yet been traced to any specific physical cause."[8] One of the reasons the medical world has been slower to recognize functional hypoglycemia is that unlike diabetes, it presents no clearcut, unmistakable symptoms, it often builds up gradually and even imperceptibly, and because of its tendency to produce more subjective psychological symptoms, it may more easily elude objective diagnosis.

To compound this problem, hypoglycemia is often noticed by the patient himself only indirectly: the general feeling of being nervous, anxious, fatigued or compulsively hungry is often regarded as "normal" in our fast-paced modern world. Unrecognized and untreated, hypoglycemia usually continues to afflict the sufferer until one of its masking complications causes him to seek diagnosis. Since these complaints number in the dozens, they are almost always treated as "independent" disorders. The experiences of one author on the subject, Dr. Stephen Gyland, illustrates the point: Dr. Gyland had himself suffered from an unexplainable list of symptoms, and had visited fourteen physicians and three famous diagnostic clinics before happening upon Dr. Harris' original 1924 paper. He then took the 5-hour GTT, and discovered that he had hypoglycemia. Dr. Gyland's case is far from unique. According to the Hypoglycemia Foundation, the average undiagnosed hypoglycemic visits twenty physicians and four psychiatrists before arriving at a diagnosis of hypoglycemia![9]

The reason for this discrepancy between how readily diabetes and hypoglycemia yield to clinical diagnosis can be traced back to their respectively more yin and more yang natures. In diabetes, glucose accumulates at the periphery, in the bloodstream, while in hypoglycemia, glucose is stored away. Similarly, diabetes as a whole shows itself at the periphery, being clearly evident and obvious, while hypoglycemia tends to squirrel itself away into the body and mind, hiding under any number of masking problems. Indeed, its wide range of commonly associated "complications" is one of the disorder's most famous features.

Mental and Neurological Problems————————————

The first organ to suffer from glucose starvation is the brain. Although only about 2 percent or 3 percent of the body's total weight, the brain uses fully 20–30 percent, ten times that proportion, of the body's glucose. (This is the reason mental work can be physically draining.) Consequently, the most dramatic and common symptoms of hypoglycemia are mental, psychological and neurological; recent X-ray studies, in fact, have recorded abnormal glucose activity in the brain in schizophrenic and manic depressive psychosis.[10]

There have been many studies that have confirmed this correlation, such as the following sampling:

A 1966 study screened a sampling of 300 psychiatric patients; 40 percent were found to be hypoglycemic.[11] Another study found a 70 percent rate of chronic hypoglycemia in diagnosed schizophrenics.[12] In a group of 220 neurotic patients with a primary complaint of anxiety or depression, 205 were found to be hypoglycemic. Subsequent work with over 700 patients continued to show the same rate of about 90 percent hypoglycemia; when treated for the blood glucose problem only, the psychiatric problems began to clear up within ten days in the majority of patients.[13] Finally, in a study in 1973, 37 patients with diagnosed reactive hypoglycemia were found to have significantly abnormal test scores on the Minnesota Multiphasic Personality Inventory (MMPI) for both hysteria and hypochondriasis.[14]

Addictions and Criminal Behavior

Adding to the problems of constant glucose starvation and general hormonal imbalance is the tendency to become partially or totally dependent on strong yin substances. In the case of alcohol and a variety of drugs, this behavior is recognized as addiction. In the case of sugared foods, soft drinks, coffee and dairy products, it is usually considered within the bounds of "normal" nourishment—but for the hypoglycemic, it bears all the hallmarks of an addiction. Actually, both diabetes and hypoglycemia tend to create addictions: in both cases, the extreme condition and lack of a stabilizing center automatically generate the need for the opposite extreme. The more yang hypoglycemic is easily addicted to strong yin (sugar, alcohol, coffee, drugs, chronic overeating, etc.), while the more yin diabetic is easily "addicted" to the powerful yang of another mammal's insulin.

Fig. 13. **Addictions are a natural attempt to seek balance for an extreme condition.**

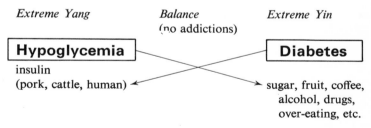

These three problems—glucose starvation of the brain, general hormonal imbalance, and chronic addictive behavior—can combine to produce a wide range of mental, emotional, psychiatric, criminal and social problems. There has been a substantial amount of research linking criminal behavior with a diet high in refined sugar refined flour, milk and "junk" foods. Again, here is a sampling of relevant studies:

(1) In a 1979 study at the San Luis Obispo Probation Department in California, Glucose Tolerance Tests revealed hypoglycemia in 16 out of the first 20 juveniles tested.[15] (2) A probation Department in a small Ohio city evaluated their client population and found that 82

percent were suffering from hypoglycemia. When the clients were treated for the disorder, their recidivism rate (rate of return to crime) dropped to 11 percent, as compared with a national rate of 66 percent.[16] (3) Linda Harding, the Child Treatment Manager at an outpatient program in Minneapolis, reported on a series of GTTs used with their clients (mostly women and their children affected by drug and alcohol abuse): over 90 percent were found to have hypoglycemia. In almost all cases, improvements were clinically documented when the clients underwent dietary improvements, including the elimination of refined sugar from their diets.[17]

Studies and trials such as these, together with growing doubts as to the effectiveness of our penal system in the deterrence of crime, have helped create a growing climate of opinion that criminal behavior should be approached and treated as a biochemical and nutritional problem.

It is often stated that it is sugar that creates hypoglycemia. Actually, sugar no more causes hypoglycemia than alcohol causes alcoholism, though it certainly is often part of the syndrome that develops. Originally, it is the lack of stabilizing complex carbohydrates (particularly whole grains) together with an overconsumption of more yang foods—eggs, poultry, cheese, meat, salt and the like—that generally causes the disorder. Sugar, alcohol, coffee, and other dietary extremes then further aggravate the imbalance.

The hypoglycemia itself creates a dim but pervasive feeling of desperation and urgency; depending upon the individual's particular dietary pattern, conditions of upbringing, social environment and other factors, this may turn inwardly, creating a worsening self-image, or outwardly. In the second case, the feelings of aggressiveness and general hostility can eventually erupt into a pattern of violent or criminal behavior. This outwardly directed explosion of pent up energies is caused by the expansive volatility of extremely yin foods like sugar, tropical fruits or drugs.

Simply eliminating the excessive yin items, therefore, can often alleviate immediately obvious symptoms; but unless the underlying cause of being attracted to those items is eliminated, the hypoglycemia will continue to worsen and eventually express itself in other ways. The same situation pertains to the problem of withdrawing from drugs and alcohol.

Alcoholism

During the Victorian era, alcoholism was widely regarded as a basic flaw in character. However, traditional societies viewed this problem as a type of mental disorder; for example, alcoholism and insanity share the same word in Sanskrit. In the modern world, it has been only in the 40 years since the end of Prohibition that addiction to alcohol has come to be regarded as a physiochemical disorder rather than a moral defect. Today there is a general consensus that nearly all alcoholics suffer from chronic hypoglycemia.[18] In fact, despite the common conception of alcoholics as weak individuals who turn to the bottle rather than face up to their own failures, alcoholics are more typically of above-average intelligence, often exceptionally talented, hard-working perfectionists at the top of their fields (a variation on the familiar "hypoglycemic personality"). In many cases, it is the obsessive cycle of drinking, spurred on by chronic hypoglycemia, that precedes the downslide in personal, family or professional life, and not the reverse.

Of course, as we would expect to find with any hypoglycemic addiction, there is a powerful emotional and spiritual component in the syndrome of alcoholism; and groups such as Alcoholics Anonymous or Alanon often deal very effectively with the problem on these levels. (In fact, many of the psychological and spiritual precepts of these two groups' philosophies bear a striking resemblance to those of macrobiotics.) Unfortunately, such approaches are limited by their lack of a complete biochemical and dietary understanding. The standard refreshment at A. A. meetings, for example, is usually coffee and doughnuts or similar snacks. Thus, though the specific abuse of alcoholism may be corrected, other equally dangerous forms of extreme substances are substituted. We must realize that alcohol itself is only the aggravating factor or catalyst here, and that the original problem is an overly yang condition (usually in a person who already has a fairly yang constitution). Once this is realized, such groups could be much more effective in achieving a complete, positive redirection towards health, and not just away from alcohol.

Drug Abuse and "Food Addictions"

Like alcohol, marijuana, cocaine, LSD, amphetamines and other mood-altering drugs work to offset the effects of low blood glucose in the short term, while in the long term badly destabilizing glucose tolerance and weakening the entire metabolism. Again, despite the widespread view that it is the social and psychological environment that leads to serious drug abuse, it is frequently a physiological imbalance that precedes the addiction, leading to chronically impaired judgment, behavioral disorders and possibly violent or criminal behavior.

The constant need to deliver a greater volume of glucose to the peripheral cells may also lead to more subtle addictions involving more socially accepted food items. The effects of sugar, coffee and tea are all similar, in that they all strongly stimulate and at the same time weaken the adrenal glands. They therefore cause an immediate rise in BG. Sugar does this more directly, by rapidly entering the blood after being broken down from disaccharides into monosaccharides, and coffee and tea more indirectly by their action on the adrenals.

Since the act of eating itself creates an initial rise in the blood's glucose (due to the automatic secretion of enteroglucagon and other hormones from the lining of the gut), hypoglycemia can also lead to a general pattern of compulsive eating. This disorder finds its most extreme expression in *bulimia*, a syndrome characterized by "binges" of staggering proportions followed by intense anxiety and self-induced vomiting; and *anorexia nervosa*, a pattern of compulsive fasting and self-starvation accompanied by profound negativism. Interestingly, both these disorders most commonly afflict young, nervous, highly success-oriented women—a description typically fitting sufferers of hypoglycemia.

Hypoglycemia and Physical Illnesses

Joslin, the famous authority on diabetes, noted on several occasions that asthma, rheumatoid arthritis and several other common disorders were extremely rare among his diabetic patients. In his book *Body, Mind and Sugar*, Dr. E. M. Abrahamson pointed out this apparent "diabetic immunity" to a variety of illnesses, suggesting that low blood glucose might be the common factor; the list included asthma, hay fever and other allergies, rheumatoid arthritis, peptic ulcer, epilepsy and alcoholism.

Observations such as these have since led to the discovery that hypoglycemia is indeed a frequent underlying condition in all these complaints: and they all tend to disappear when hyperglycemia appears, due either to the late onset of diabetes or to the administration of diabetogenic drugs. (Most of the drugs routinely prescribed for these and other illness have the effect of raising blood glucose levels.) For example, it is common for patients with asthma or rheumatoid arthritis to find to their delight that around the age of forty or fifty, their symptoms disappear . . . only to find that they have begun to develop Type II diabetes.

Responding to the criticism that the causal role of hypoglycemia in these disorders has not been clinically proven, Dr. Abrahamson replies,

". . . our concern as to whether [hypoglycemia] is cause or effect is groundless. . . . We like to imagine a well-ordered state of affairs in which each action is produced by some antecedent cause and in turn produces its own effect. But . . . Nature does not function in this manner. In all cases of undesirable functioning of the body accompanied by low blood sugar, the only condition of the body that is vulnerable to therapy of a simple nature is the level of the blood glucose . . . ."[19]

Each of these disorders arises through a different mechanism, yet they are all variations of the hypoglycemic pattern: accumulating excess and stagnated functions, an overly yang condition in general, and often an overcompensating indulgence in strong yin substances which only complicates the problem. The genesis of epilepsy, for example, is similar to that of hypoglycemic psychological problems, except that it is the rear portion of the brain, controlling more unconscious and motor activities, that is the site of sensitivity. The intake of strong yin, such as beer, wine or sugared drinks, expands the nerve tissues in this region and creates pressure leading to abnormal nerve functioning and seizure. Asthma, allergies, arthritis and others are all symptoms of accumulations in the respiratory, digestive, skeletal and other systems.

Regarding stomach ulcers, it is interesting to note that injecting insulin is a common method of diagnosing digestive activity. In normal health, an increased level of insulin causes the stomach to vigorously secrete its acid digestive juices. A chronically low level of insulin antagonists, therefore, can easily lead to hypersecretion of these acids and eventually to ulcer.

Hypoglycemia as a Precursor to Diabetes

Ironically, though hypoglycemia is opposite to diabetes in so many respects, one of its most widespread life-threatening complications is that it often leads to diabetes itself. This apparent contradiction is easily understood in terms of yin and yang. The overly yang condition of hypoglycemia causes a powerful attraction to strongly yin foods, drinks and drugs; in many cases, this can eventually lead from one extreme, hypoglycemia, to the other, diabetes.

Yin and Yang and the GTT

The most fascinating aspect of the common Oral Glucose Tolerance Test is that it illustrates fairly accurately the balance of yang and yin forces in an individual's condition. A very high or steeply upward line reveals the influence of very strong expanding (yin and upward) energy, while a very low or sharply falling line indicates more descending, yang energy. This tends to correlate not only with the foods and eating patterns that cause those fluctuations in BG, but also with personality and behavioral traits, mental outlook, voice patterns, and even the person's physical patterns of movement and gesturing.

For example, we can draw the following conclusions about the diets of the persons whose GTT profiles are shown in Figure 14:

Fig. 14.   Examples of the OGTT (Oral Glucose Tolerance Test).

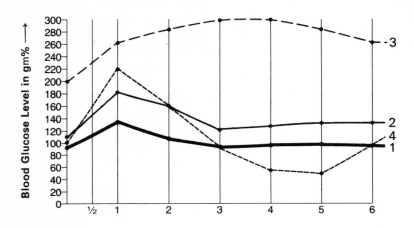

Fig. 14-A.   Hours after Administering Oral Glucose Load ⟶

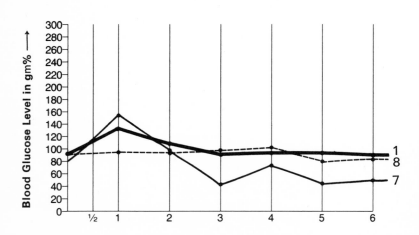

Fig. 14-B.   Hours after Administering Oral Glucose Load ⟶

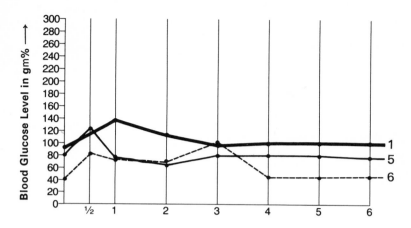

Fig. 14–C. Hours after Administering Oral Glucose Load ⟶

1. Normal
2. Mild Diabetes. Same shape as #1, but higher on the graph. May be Type II.
3. Severe Diabetes. Different shape altogether: probably Type I.
4. "Dysinsulinism." Extremes of both yin and yang; renal threshold of 180 mg% is passed (indicating diabetes), yet a drop of over 120 mg% in just 2 hours also indicates severe hypoglycemia.
5. Mild Hypoglycemia. Same shape as #1; may sometimes be considered "normal," and may or may not have hypoglycemic symptoms.

6. Severe Hypoglycemia. Never really reaches an adequate BG level; note the unusual high at the third hour—may be due to adrenals; overall more yang, anxious personality.
7. Severe Hypoglycemia. Extremes of both yin and yang, but more yang than #4.
8. "Flat Curve" Hypoglycemia. Although all BG values are well within "normal" range, the graph's shape is abnormal, showing almost no response to ingested glucose load; very dull, yang, undramatic personality.

• Number Four and Number Seven (dysinsulinism): chaotic eating patterns, including big extremes of both yin and yang. However, Number Seven's diet contains more volume of salt and animal foods, while Number Four's includes more sugar, fruit and possibly drugs or stimulants. We would also expect a correspondingly chaotic pattern of mood swings and behavioral changes, as well as more exaggerated vocal and possibly facial mannerisms.

- Number Two (Type II diabetes) and Number Five (mild hypoglycemia): in contrast to Number Four and Number Seven, more regular or consistent eating habits; but over time the overly yin quality of Number Two's diet and overly yang quality of Number Five's have gradually thrown their metabolisms off balance.
- Number Three (Type I diabetes): very yin diet.
- Number Six (severe hypoglycemia): overall very heavy, yang diet, but with a wide variety and some more strongly yin items such as sugared coffee, wine or fruit juices.
- Number Eight ("Flat Curve" hypoglycemia): very consistent, repetitive eating habits, probably consisting of eggs, meats, bread, potatoes and no strong yin foods, only salads and perhaps a regular moderate serving of fruit, beer or wine.

While the personalities of Number Four and Number Seven are probably the most dramatic and dynamic of the eight, that of Number Eight is just the opposite. The latter curve ("Flat Curve") reveals someone whose life is given to monotonous, routine work—often a factory worker, housewife or lower echelon businessman—who lacks a sense of zest and suffers from chronic boredom, fatigue, and lack of sexual appetite.[20]

This discussion is presented to illustrate the remarkably practical, adaptable nature of yin and yang as a means of assessing the significance of virtually any data or details of observation. However, the process of actually taking a GTT itself is often quite stressful, as it involves a fast followed by the consumption of pure glucose, and it is not recommended in every case.

What is the Scope of Hypoglycemia?

From this brief survey of some of the common hypoglycemic complications, it is clear that there exists a considerable range of individual variation in just how a carbohydrate metabolism problem may manifest itself—in fact, it is probable that no two cases are exactly alike. Further, it is apparent that the sheer scope of the disorder is vast, indeed.

How many people suffer from hypoglycemia? Conservative estimates place the incidence at between 10 percent and 25 percent of the population[2]; but many authorities feel the figure is far higher. As in the case of diabetes, the impact of the disorder's associated complications is far greater than that caused directly by hypoglycemia itself. Again, there is no way to directly assess these damages, but considering the close relationship of hypoglycemia to problems such as alcoholism, drug abuse and other addictions, chronic depression and other psychiatric problems, violent crime, rheumatoid arthritis and allergies (to name the most prominent handful), its repercussions on the individual sufferers and on society at large must certainly be seen as severe.

A public health survey conducted by the U.S. Department of Health, Education and Welfare in 1966–67 found 66,000 cases of hypoglycemia reported out of the 134,000 individuals interviewed, representing a startling 49.2 percent.[3] It is interesting that the language of the survey itself did not mention hypoglycemia at all in its questions; and since the term was not nearly as well known in 1967 as it is today, it seems likely that even this may today be well below the mark. Unfortunately, it is difficult to find any authoritative figures from more recent sources; but my experiences with thousands of individuals suggests that as many as 75 percent of the general population in modern cultures—3 out of every 4 persons—suffer from some degree of chronically low or unstable blood glucose.

Ironically, though official figures put diabetes as the seventh leading cause of death, if we total up the possible annual damages from hypoglycemia in mortality, loss of property and income, medical expenses and the toll of human suffering, the impact of hypoglycemia may be even more extensive than that of its sister disease! For example, though heart disease and cancer are commonly known to be our first and second leading cause of death, anxiety and depression (usually involving hypoglycemia) as clinical syndromes outrank all other diagnosed health problems in general medicine. According to one expert, "the incidence [of these two problems] in the U.S. today is not known. Even an estimate would be nothing more than a guess."[21]

Taken as a whole, we may consider carbohydrate metabolism disorders —diabetes and hypoglycemia and all their attendant complications—as our primary leading threat to health. And this is not surprising: these problems are simply a direct reflection of our departure from the traditional ways of eating we have so drastically disavowed.

[1]   Cahill's *Encyclopaedia of Medicine*, entry under "Hypoglycemia."
[2]   Light, p. 8.
[3]   Dr. Carlton Fredericks, quoted in Airola, p. 15.
[4]   Osterritter, p. 133.
[5]   Light, p. 6 ff.
[6]   Light, p. 7.
[7]   *Symptoms*. Sigmund S. Miller, ed., Avon Books, NY 1978, p. 484.
[8]   Weller, p. 1, p. 9.
[9]   Dufty, p. 91.
[10]   *Newsweek*, "Scanning the Human Mind," Sept. 29, 1980, p. 63.
[11]   Saltzer, H. M., M. D., "Relative Hypoglycemia as a Cause of Neuropsychiatric Illness," *Journal of the National Medical Association*, Jan. 1966, Vol. 58, No. 1, p. 12.
[12]   Ibid., p. 27.
[13]   Abrahamson, p. 109.

[14] Anthony, et al., "Personality Disorder in Reactive Hypoglycemia, *Diabetes*, 22: 664, 1973.

[15] Schauss, p. 12.

[16] McQuire, D., "Crime Linked with Dietary Habits," *Rochester Democrat & Chronicle*, Sept. 27, 1979, p. 1C.

[17] Schauss, p. 17.

[18] Osterritter, p. 131.

[19] Abrahamson, p. 177–178.

[20] See Airola, p. 32 and Abrahamson, pp. 111–126.

[21] Osterritter. p. 127.

4. The Conventional Dietary Approach ▬▬▬▬

Considering the lack of a clear consensus on the cause of diabetes, it is not surprising that there has been considerable debate over how to best treat the disease. Prior to the insulin era, modification of diet was the primary therapy in the management of diabetes. Unfortunately, the nature of the disease and of diet itself were so poorly understood that the diets prescribed often did more harm than good—in the words of Dr. Abrahamson, "a vivid example of the flounderings of medicine in the pursuit of knowledge."[1]

The Conventional Diabetes Diet ▬▬▬▬▬▬▬▬▬▬▬▬

The logic of the classical dietary model was simple: since diabetics have excess sugar in their urine, they should avoid carbohydrates as completely as possible. It is impractical to increase protein intake beyond a certain level, so the balance of daily calories was to be made up with an increased intake of fat. This basic concept was advanced in 1796 by the British physician John Rollo, and has been the basis of most diabetic diets up until the last ten or fifteen years. The most obvious problem with the classic low-carbohydrate, high-fat diet was its extreme unpalatability. Many patients were simply unable to eat the large proportions of animal fat and protein it required, and success with the diets was limited.[2]

In 1928, the renowned diabetologist Dr. Elliot Joslin of the world-famous Boston Diabetes Clinic startled the medical world by suggesting that the high fat diets prescribed to help improve diabetics' conditions may have actually been the primary cause of diabetic cardiovascular complications.[3] By this time the routine use of insulin had reduced the apparent need to follow such strict dietary control anyway, and the medical profession responded to Dr. Joslin's warning by relaxing the standard recommendations. Eventually, in the early 1970s, diabetics were told they could eat a "free diet" resembling non-diabetics' normal eating patterns as closely as possible.[4]

The problem with this advice was that what constituted the prevailing "normal" diet had by now changed drastically, with a considerable increase in fats, refined sugars and animal foods, and a correspondingly steep decrease in complex carbohydrates. By traditional standards, the normal diet of 1973 was already a high-fat, low-carbohydrate diet! And in the meantime, a sizable body of evidence had appeared implicating these dietary changes in the cause of diabetes, as well as of cardiovascular illnesses and other leading health problems.

As early as 1935, it had been shown that the diets diabetics followed prior to developing the disease were not high in starch, but were high in fat. One researcher pointed out that populations whose diets consisted primarily of carbohydrates, such as the Chinese and Japanese, had a very low incidence of diabetes, while those with the highest diabetes rates (including Jewish and Italian communities) consumed a great deal of animal fat and vegetable oils.[5] (Diabetics have also been found to eat significantly more food in general than non-diabetics.)[6]

Further epidemiological evidence supports this view. The incidence of heart attack and stroke in diabetics, for example, is five times higher in America than in Japan (where much less fat is consumed), while diabetic gangrene is 100 times more common.[7] And nearly a decade earlier two Viennese doctors, Adlesberg and Porges, had made the revolutionary discovery that fat restriction yielded far better results in the treatment of diabetes than carbohydrate restriction.[8]

While the case against fat was mounting, the evidence indicting refined sugar had been accumulating for decades. An entry for diabetes mellitus in the 1911 *Encyclopedia Britannica* reads: "The excessive use of sugar as a food is usually considered one of the causes of the disease."[9] While there are no early figures available for sugar consumption in the United States, such statistics do exist for Denmark, which was the leading European consumer of sugar prior to World War II. The comparison of increase in annual per capita sugar intake and diabetes death rates is revealing:

	lbs sugar (per person per year)	diabetes deaths (per 100,000 pop.)
1880	29	1.8
1911	82	8
1936	113	18.9

(from *Sugar Blues*, p. 79.)

The sharp drop in diabetes rates in European countries during both World Wars, when wartime food rations drastically cut back the civilian intake of both fat and sugar, is another piece of evidence often cited in the case for dietary origins of the disease.

Despite the growing wealth of evidence, though, the classical carbohydrate restriction model remained the mainstay of dietary policy throughout much of the twentieth century—and the role of diet in both treatment and prevention has largely fallen under the shadow of more spectacular directions in diabetes research and development. With the advent of insulin therapy in 1921, the new direction towards pharmaceutical "control" also signaled a shift away from research on the role of diet and nutrition. In 1929, seeing this alarming trend, the "father" of insulin therapy, Banting himself, "tried to tell us that his discovery was merely a palliative, not a cure, and that the way to prevent diabetes was to cut down on 'dangerous' sugar bingeing."[10] He also pointed out that "in the U.S., the incidence of diabetes has increased proportionately with the per capita consumption of [refined] sugar."[11]

These and other similar warnings went unheeded, however, and up until the last ten or fifteen years the emphasis in research and development of treatments for diabetes has been decidedly on newer types of insulin, oral drugs, and several recent technological innovations such as bio-engineering and artificial organ design.

The Conventional Approach to Hypoglycemia

Most approaches to the treatment of hypoglycemia are dietary programs more or less based on the diet plan first devised by the founding pioneer of hypoglycemia research. The "Seale Harris Diet" is essentially a high-protein, high-fat, low-carbohydrate regimen organized around the idea that refined carbohydrates (as well as coffee and other stimulants) are the cause of the disorder. Refined carbohydrates, starchy foods, coffee, alcohol and other similarly yin items are strictly avoided, and carbohydrates in general are carefully limited. (As in the field of diabetes treatment, there are practitioners who have recommended dietary approaches more closely resembling that of macrobiotics, notably Paavo Airola in his book *Hypoglycemia: A Better Approach*. On the whole, though, the Seale Harris model still represents the mainstream of nutritional thinking on this question.)

While it is of course highly advisable to avoid these more yin foods, the Harris diet is unfortunate in its emphasis on animal foods and its sparse use of even complex carbohydrates. In fact, this approach is as inappropriate, though far more intelligently intended, as the physician's simplistic suggestion to eat more sugar. It is exactly these foods—meats, eggs, poultry and dairy products—that originally caused the disorder!

Curiously, this approach often produces a rapid though temporary relief of the worst symptoms. Eliminating the extremely yin items naturally reduces the extreme fluctuation of BG. Furthermore, the high protein nature of the diet starves the body of dietary glucose, forcing the liver and adrenals to increase their efforts to draw on the body's stores for fuel. (This is the reason high-protein diets are sometimes used for weight reduction.) At the same time, though, both the liver and kidneys are put under tremendous strain to try and neutralize the toxic effects of such a diet.

Before long, the accumulations of animal fat and protein and the stagnation of the liver and adrenals are all greater than ever. The lack of complex carbohydrates, moreover, destabilizes the body's capacity to manage its BG level—and the hypoglycemic condition, after appearing to improve for a brief period, becomes more solidly entrenched than when the treatment began.

This approach clearly illustrates the dangers of approaching a problem analytically, without a larger, more embracing perspective. There are four major misconceptions operating here:

1. It is not an excess of carbohydrate but the lack of carbohydrate that leads to hypoglycemia.
2. A high-animal food diet does not improve but greatly worsens the condition.
3. The same general diet plan is recommended for both diabetes and hypoglycemia; yet these are opposite conditions, and naturally should be approached with different diets.
4. Finally, the dietary pattern recommended is a radical departure from most traditional diets—yet most people eating in that traditional way did not experience either disorder nearly as much as modern people.

In addition to diet, various supplements are often prescribed for hypoglycemia, including synthetic or "natural" vitamins, minerals, enzymes and hormone extracts, particularly adrenal cortex hormones. However, the use of such special supplements is unnecessary at best (except in cases where the surgical removal or irradiation of a gland necessitates the use of a glandular supplement) and dangerous at worst.

The thinking involved in relying upon vitamin, mineral and enzyme supplements is somewhat backwards—it was the excessive refining and processing of foods that first led to the practice of artificially extracting nutrients and using them as supplements. The most sensible course of action is to avoid this kind of adulteration in the first place, and instead use the whole natural food itself, with all its nutrients intact. The idea of adding bran to white bread, for example, is patently absurd. If we need the bran, why remove it in the first place? The sheer complexity of properly calculating all our individual needs for each known micronutrient also makes the task of consuming them piecemeal virtually impossible. Also, since the body is not equipped to handle these micronutrients in such a concentrated, extracted form (any more than it is able to cope with refined sugar), their use can place a significant strain on the liver, kidneys and other protective organs.

Artificially administered hormones, like vitamin supplements, may overstimulate the organism and tax its excretory functions. Further, their regular use can foster a dependency in the glands they are intended to aid. Generally, it is advisable to avoid such supplements whenever possible. Even in cases where they must be used, due to glandular damage or dysfunction, it is often possible to gradually reduce their dosage, and in some cases even eliminate them, as the body regains its natural strength and adaptability.

New Developments in Diet

In the mid-1970's, the medical and scientific world was rocked by a revolution in the medical status of diet and nutrition. Within the span of half a decade, several dozen reports from leading scientific and governmental agencies appeared, drawing a clear link between modern patterns of disease and diet. The new ground was first broken in the appropriately historical bi-centennial year of 1976 with the U. S. Senate Nutrition Sub-Committee report *Dietary Goals for the United States*, chaired by Senator McGovern:

"... there is a great deal of evidence, and it continues to accumulate, which strongly implicates and in some cases proves that the major causes of death and disability in the United States are related to the diet we eat ...." (Dr. Mark Hegsted, in *Dietary Goals for the U.S.*)

Examples cited included heart disease, several major types of cancer, obesity, and diabetes. The report went on to recommend a substantial return to more traditional eating patterns, including a decreased consumption of fat, cholesterol, sugar and refined or highly processed foods, and a parallel increase in complex carbohydrate foods such as whole grains, fresh vegetables and fruits. In reference to diabetes, the report concluded that such dietary changes would result in 50 percent of cases being improved or prevented entirely.[12] Similar findings and recommendations were soon echoed in reports and guidelines from the U.S. Surgeon General, the American Heart Association, the American Society for Clinical Nutrition, the U. S. Department of Agriculture and Department of Health, Education and Welfare, the National Research Council and many others in the United States and abroad.

Within this dramatically broad-based climate of national dietary self-reflection, the American Diabetes Association issued a new set of guidelines in 1979 that amounted to a reversal of earlier policies.

"It is recognized that the field of nutrition is a dynamic science. As new facts emerge and concepts change, the nutritional recommendations for diabetic and nondiabetic persons will continue to undergo evolution and modification . . . . In general, some liberalization in carbohydrate intake is recommended, preferably as complex carbohydrate . . . and as a replacement for some of the fat." (From the special report *Principles of Nutrition and Dietary Recommendations for Individuals with Diabetes Mellitus: 1979*, American Diabetes Association.)

The report went on to recommend that carbohydrate should comprise fully 50–60 percent of the diet, with only 20–38 percent fat; that saturated fats should be decreased to under 10 percent at maximum, with the balance of fats from unsaturated sources; that foods containing cholesterol, disaccharides, refined carbohydrate or special high-protein preparations should be avoided; and that vegetarian or semi-vegetarian programs, if nutritionally balanced, were acceptable as diabetic diets. A new era in diabetic dietary management had begun.

Advances in the Past Decade

One of the most respected pioneers of this new dietary direction is Dr. James Anderson, a professor of medicine and clinical nutrition who currently directs a diabetes program at the Veterans Administration Hospital in Lexington, Kentucky. Anderson advocates a high-carbohydrate, high-fiber diet (HCF), containing approximately 75 percent of calories from high-fiber complex carbohydrates, 16 percent from protein and only 9 percent from fat (roughly similar to the nutritional breakdown of an average macrobiotic diet). In a book written for the public, he says that "in many ways, the high-fiber diet plans we have devised are the opposite of the traditional diabetic diets," pointing out that there were never any scientific experiments carried out to support the older theory of carbohydrate restriction.[13]

In 1975, Anderson and his colleagues tested the HCF diet on thirteen diabetic men, aged 30–35, all of whom were at that time following a diet of approximately 43 percent carbohydrate, 23 percent protein and 34 percent fat. The results were impressive: five of the men taking oral hypoglycemics were able to discontinue them, four more were able to stop their insulin therapies, and all of the others had shown some reduction in blood glucose and cholesterol levels. Speaking of these and subsequent trials, Anderson declares that "Every patient that we have treated with the HCF diet has gained some improvement in his or her diabetes . . . we have been able to discontinue insulin therapy in 18 out of 20 patients taking less than 25 units per day [and in 8 out of 15 taking 25–40 units per day] . . . [the HCF diets] lower insulin needs by an average of 25 percent."[14]

Anderson cites supporting studies from Oxford, San Diego and Denmark in his claim that his HCF dietary concept has been widely recognized in nutritional circles. He also suggests that an even greater decrease of animal fats and cholesterol would improve the effectiveness of the HCF diet still further; and that nondiabetics as well stand to gain considerable health benefits from this type of program.

In a recent study of a program similar to Anderson's, Hans Diehl and Don Mannerberg evaluated the progress of 54 diabetic patients in a 4-week program at Nathan Pritikin's famous Longevity Center in Santa Monica, California. The diet followed in Pritikin's program was a largely vegetarian (small amounts of fish and white meat were allowed), HCF-type diet including 70 percent complex carbohydrates, no refined sugars, restricted refined starches and negligible amounts of cholesterol. Prior to admission into the program, 32 patients were taking oral hypoglycemics, and the other 22 were using insulin. At the conclusion of the four weeks, only 6 of the original 32 were still taking the oral drugs, fully one-half of the insulin-taking patients had completely ceased their insulin therapy and achieved normal blood glucose levels, and most of the other eleven insulin-takers had decreased their requirements.[15]

The National Heart and Diabetes Treatment Institute is another program similar to Anderson's and Pritikin's, run by Dr. Julian Whitaker in Huntingdon Beach, California. Using a largely vegetarian HCF-type diet together with regular exercise and vitamin/mineral supplementation, Whitaker reports that over half the insulin-dependent diabetics enrolled in his program have been able to discontinue their insulin therapy. His diet, which relies heavily on whole grains and vegetables, is quite similar to Pritikin's (the two once worked together), the primary difference being that Whitaker allows no meat at all and very little of any other animal source foods.[16]

The Importance of Dietary Fiber

In addition to complex carbohydrates and the avoidance or fats and sugars, dietary fiber has emerged as a key factor in controlling or avoiding diabetes. In their book *Western Diseases: Their Emergence and Prevention*, Drs. Denis Burkitt and Hugh Trowell compared diet and disease patterns of the developed countries with those of dozens of rural populations, notably African communities. Their studies suggested that a diet high in natural fibers may prevent obesity and help protect against colon cancer, heart disease, strokes and diabetes. Recently, both human and laboratory studies have shown that certain types of fiber—particularly soluble fibers such as the gums found in lentils, dried beans and whole oats—help regulate the intestinal absorption of nutrients and thereby reduce insulin requirements. In one study, a breakfast containing lentils was found to produce a flatter (more normal) BG response to both the breakfast itself and the following lunch. Conversely, other studies have shown that while a higher fat food can slow absorption of the carbohydrates it accompanies, it will impair the glucose response of the following meal.

From a commonsense perspective, none of these findings should surprise us at all. It stands to reason that the fibers plants create to build their stored glucose fuels into firm structures are an essential part of our nourishment. If we take only the stored fuel without the structural member that gives it form, it is only natural that we will eventually become unable to ˙.se those fuels properly, and our own structures will deteriorate. If ˇ e grow lax in our physiological chores of breaking down naturally complex carbohydrates for fuel and building up needed body fats out of plant foods, and instead relegate these tasks to sugar refineries and tamed animals, it is only reasonable to expect that our metabolisms will weaken as surely as over-use of escalators produces flabby legs. The laboratory methods of science have finally caught up with and confirmed the ages-old folk wisdom: we are not only what we eat, but also how we digest and metabolize what we eat.

Food Exchanges Versus the "Glycemic Index"———

By the 1980's the conventional approach to diabetic diets had been almost totally invalidated by science. The final blow came in 1983, when the universally accepted concept of carbohydrate "food exchanges" crumbled under the weight of several startling new studies. The idea of food exchanges, like that of the high-fat, low-starch diets, was a simple one. Science had earlier made the error of assuming that all carbohydrates (whether simple or complex) had similar effects on the body, which had led to the unfortunate exclusion of such foods as grains because they were "sugars." Having come to recognize the world of difference between simple and complex carbohydrates, the prevailing view arose that at least within these two categories, foods had a roughly parallel effect. Thus, by following a carbohydrate exchange list, diabetics could begin from one prototype menu and vary it by substituting, for example, potatoes for rice or whole wheat bread for corn.

This assumption points out the Achilles' heel of the modern scientific method—that the behaviors of unique life phenomena can be mechanically reduced to numerical equivalents for measurement and manipulation. The carbohydrate exchange concept, however, had never been experimentally confirmed; and when two Denver, Colorado researchers, Phyllis Crapo and her husband, diabetologist Jerrold Olefsky, decided to risk simply proving the obvious by actually testing the theory, their results hit that Achilles' heel with a devastating bulls-eye.[17]

What Crapo and Olefsky found was that every different food tested produced a unique glycemic response, and the pattern of these responses showed no resemblance to theoretical predictions whatsoever. Rice, for example, produced a flat glucose response, while potatoes elicited the kind of rapid glucose reaction one would expect from a load of pure glucose— Olefsky exclaimed that "potatoes are like candy as far as a diabetic is concerned."[18] From the standpoint of yin and yang, this result is easily explained and could have been easily predicted: potatoes are extremely yin and in fact are usually excluded in macrobiotic dietary recommendations. Their tests and others carried out soon afterward in Toronto and Oxford produced quite a few surprises:

- lentils and beans yielded very low glycemic responses (confirming the earlier studies on soluble fibers); however,
- ice cream and yogurt also produced extremely low responses (thought to be due to the slower absorption caused by their higher fat content);
- bread and corn both produced sharper responses than rice; buckwheat, in turn, was rated even better than rice in this respect (on the scale of yin and yang, corn is the most yin grain, while buckwheat is the most yang);
- noodles provoked much less of a glycemic reaction than breads; yet breads taken together with beans resulted in the low reaction characteristic of beans (far lower than noodles) rather than the high response of bread alone;
- the texture of foods effected their glycemic rating, a wetter, creamier texture producing a faster rise in glucose; for example, "rice slurry" and pureed apples both caused a more rapid response than rice grains and whole apple.

These sensational findings rapidly received considerable publicity, leading to the hasty conclusion on the part of many that the lower on the "glycemic index" a food rated, the better it was for diabetics. If true, this would mean that ice cream and potato chips were as good as lentils and superior to brown rice and cooked carrots. Other researchers were quick to point out that this was a serious oversimplification: other factors would need to be integrated with the new glycemic index before the effects of specific foods could be properly reassessed. Studies had already shown, for example, that although adding fat to carbohydrate produced a flatter glucose curve by slowing absorption, it had no such effect on the person's actual insulin response; moreover, high-fat low-glycemic-index foods such as buttered potatoes, potato chips or ice cream actually impaired glucose tolerance in the subsequent meal.[19]

Crapo herself summed up the implications of these new findings succinctly: "What happens when we eat food is much more complex than anyone thought."[20] Another researcher involved in the studies suggested that overall, "these findings point us in the direction of more primitive diets having great merits."[21] Meanwhile, the president of the American Diabetes Association, Irving Spratt, declared that the organization was considering reworking the existing exchange lists to reflect the new research.[22]

Today, the scientific viewpoint of diet's role in diabetes stands at a new threshold. The conventional dietary understanding has proven wholly inadequate, and the new nutrition emerging is as bewilderingly different from the old views as modern sub-particle physics is from Newton's laws of motion. Every evidence points to a return to a more traditional, "primitive" diet; yet the conventional methods of classifying foods no longer seem equal to the task of designing such a diet. What is still clearly lacking is a comprehensive, systematic approach, far beyond the conventional descriptions of nutrition, for evaluating individual foods and their effects on individual human health. To fill this gap, we can expect that the next decade will see a strong interest rekindling in the viewpoints of ancient dietary medicine, as revived under the aegis of macrobiotics: for this comprehensive view is precisely what the macrobiotic approach and the study of yin and yang provide.

---

[1] Abrahamson, p. 20.
[2] Abrahamson, p. 20–21, 24–26; *EWJ*, p. 27–28.
[3] Anderson, p. 90.
[4] 1973 *Encyclopedia Britannica*, quoted in *EWJ*.
[5] Abrahamson, p. 28–29.
[6] Davidson, et al., p. 348.
[7] Anderson, p. 91.
[8] Abrahamson, p. 28.
[9] Quoted in Dufty, p. 80.
[10] Dufty, p. 82.
[11] F. G. Banting, *Strength and Health*. May–June, 1972. Quoted in Dufty, p. 82.
[12] *Dietary Goals*, p. 73.
[13] Anderson, p. 90.
[14] Anderson, p. 97–98.
[15] Trowell, p. 396 ff.

[16] *Nutrition for the Prevention and Treatment of Heart Disease, Diabetes and Hypertension*, Julian Whitaker, M. D., National Heart and Diabetes Treatment Institute, Ca., 1982.

[17] *Nutrition Action*, Sept. 1983, Center for Science and the Public Interest, Washington D. C., p. 8–11; *Science*, April 29, 1983, p. 487–488.

[18] *Science*, op cit, p. 487.

[19] Letter from Kerin O'Dea, Dept. of Medicine, University of Melbourne, printed in *Science*, July 15, 1983.

[20] *Science*, April 29, 1983. p. 487.

[21] David Jenkins of the University of Toronto, *EWJ* p. 29.

[22] *Science*, op cit.

5. The Macrobiotic Approach to Diabetes and Hypoglycemia ━━━━━━━━

The following guidelines represent a standard or average macrobiotic way of eating, and can be safely followed by anyone already in generally good health to avoid the risk of developing diabetes, hypoglycemia or any of the many other ills prevalent in modern life. At the same time, it should be remembered that there is no one diet that is perfect for everyone. In fact, this general pattern should be freely varied and adjusted to suit variations in climate, season, past eating habits, one's individual condition and other factors. A brief discussion of some of these factors is presented in the companion volume *Diabetes and Hypoglycemia* in the *Macrobiotic Food and Cooking Series*.

These guidelines are followed by a section on how to tailor dietary adjustments more specifically to suit the needs of those with an already developed diabetic or hypoglycemic condition. In the case of persons who have a particular disorder, it is recommended that these guidelines be followed under the supervision of a qualified macrobiotic counselor as well as an appropriate medical or nutritional health professional. It is also strongly suggested that the reader pursue a more complete and practical understanding of these guidelines by attending qualified macrobiotic cooking courses. A list of appropriate Resources appears in the Appendix.

These guidelines are presented in terms of percent of total daily volume eaten. It is not necessary to weigh or measure precisely the quantity of each food or portion; an approximate comparison of serving size is sufficient. Whole grains can be the principal dish (at least fifty percent) at each meal, with vegetables as the primary side dish, though it is not necessary to include all side dish categories (soup, beans, etc.) at each meal. The total volume eaten may vary considerably from person to person and from day to day, and need not be fixed; but the proper relative proportions of different food categories, regardless of total volume, should be maintained.

WHOLE GRAINS: At least one half (fifty to sixty percent) of daily food may be cooked whole grains and their products. The majority of grains may be eaten in whole form, with a lesser amount consumed as flour, cracked or otherwise processed grains. Grains may be cooked 45–55 minutes and seasoned with a pinch of natural (unrefined) seasalt; brown rice and other whole grains are best prepared in a stainless steel or enamel/

steel pressure-cooker. *Grains for daily or regular use* include: brown rice (short or medium grain); barley; millet; whole oats; whole wheat berries; whole rye; whole corn; buckwheat; Job's Tears ("pearl barley" or *hato mugi*). *Grains for occasional use* include: sweet brown rice and *mochi* (pounded sweet brown rice dumpling); long grain brown rice; whole-grain noodles such as *udon* (Japanese whole-wheat noodles), *soba* (buckwheat noodles) and whole-wheat pasta; unleavened or natural sourdough whole-wheat or rye bread, traditionally prepared flat breads, tortillas or chapati; bulgur, cracked wheat and cracked rye; steel-cut ("Scotch") or rolled oats; corn grits and meal; couscous; *seitan* (wheat gluten cutlet) or *fu* (puffed wheat gluten).

SOUP: One or two cups or bowls of soup (about five percent of total volume) may be consumed daily; these may contain a variety of ingredients, including seasonal vegetables, sea vegetables (particularly *kombu* or *wakame*), and occasionally grains or beans, and should be mildly seasoned with naturally processed *miso* or *tamari* soy sauce (also known as *shoyu*). Barley (*mugi*) *miso*, soybean (*hatcho*) *miso* and brown rice (*genmai*) *miso* are the most suitable varieties for daily use.

VEGETABLES: Approximately one quarter to one third of each meal may include fresh vegetables prepared in a variety of ways, including steaming, boiling, simmering, sautéing and others, including both dishes cooked a shorter time (from three to fifteen minutes) and with a fresher taste, and dishes cooked a longer time (fifteen to forty-five minutes) and with a heartier taste. The proportion of these two general styles can be varied with the season and climate, the fresher dishes being especially suited to hotter environments and the heartier dishes being more suitable for colder environments. In addition, up to one third of vegetables dishes may be eaten as parboiled, pressed or raw salads and as unspiced natural pickles. *Vegetables for daily or regular use* include:

1.   Root and stem vegetables: burdock, carrot, *daikon* (long white) radish (fresh and dried), dandelion root, lotus root (fresh and dried), onion, parsnip, radish, rutabaga, salsify, turnip.
2.   Ground vegetables: cauliflower, hard squashes (acorn, buttercup, butternut, hubbard, etc.), pumpkin and Hokkaido pumpkin.
3.   Green and white leafy vegetables: broccoli, brussel sprouts, bok choy, green cabbage, carrot tops, Chinese cabbage, chives, collard greens, *daikon* greens, dandelion greens, kale, leeks, mustard greens, *nappa*, parsley, scallion, turnip greens, watercress.

Vegetables for occasional use include: celery, cucumber, endive, escarole, fresh beans (string beans, snap beans, wax or yellow beans, etc.), green peas, Chinese snow peas, *jinenjo* (mountain potato), kohlrabi, lettuce, mushrooms, *shiitake* mushrooms, red cabbage, soft squashes (patty pan, summer squash and zucchini), Swiss chard.

Fig. 15.   The standard macrobiotic diet.

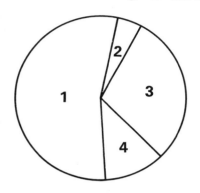

1. 50–60% whole unrefined cereal grains.
2. 5% naturally seasoned soups.
3. 25–30% fresh vegetables.
4. 10–15% beans, sea vegetables and supplementary foods. Plus appropriate volumes of mild beverages.

BEANS AND SEA VEGETABLES: About five to ten percent of daily food may include cooked beans and bean products as an additional protein source, and a smaller quantity of cooked sea vegetables as an additional source of minerals and vitamins. This may amount to one moderate serving of beans daily or often, and up to several tablespoons of sea vegetables daily. Beans are best well-cooked and seasoned moderately with seasalt, *miso* or *tamari* soy sauce. Sea vegetables may be used as ingredients in other dishes (such as soups, beans or vegetables dishes), as table condiments, or several times per week as side dishes, seasoned moderately with *tamari* soy sauce and/or a mild grain vinegar such as brown rice vinegar.

Beans for daily or regular use include: *azuki* (small red) beans, brown lentils, chick peas (garbanzo beans); soybean products such as *tofu* (fresh or dried), *tempeh* or *natto* may also be included on a regular basis.

Beans for occasional use include: black-eyed peas, black (turtle) beans, black soybeans, great northern beans, kidney beans, lima beans, navy beans, split peas and whole dried peas.

All edible sea vegetables are suitable for *daily or regular use*, including: agar-agar or *kanten* (as a gelatin for molds), *arame* (as a side dish), dulse, *hijiki* (as a side dish), Irish moss, *kombu* (for soup stocks, with beans or vegetable dishes, as condiment), *mekabu* (as a side dish), *nori* (as a garnish, condiment or as a coating over rice balls or *sushi*), *wakame* (as a side dish, in soups or as condiment).

SUPPLEMENTARY FOODS: *Seafood.* Depending upon your condition
and desire, you may include a moderate volume of white-meat, non-fatty
fish up to several times per week, preferably prepared without oil (broiled,
boiled, steamed or as soup) and served together with a larger volume of
freshly steamed or boiled leafy vegetables. *Suitable varieties include:*
flounder, sole, halibut, cod, schrod, haddock, trout, clams, oysters, scal-
lops, shrimp and others. Whole dried small fish, called *chirimen* or *chuba
iriko,* may be used occasionally as a seasoning or condiment.

Seeds and Nuts: A small volume of seeds may be used daily or often,
either lightly roasted and seasoned with seasalt or *tamari* and eaten as a
snack or used as condiments or in dishes. *Suitable varieties* include: sesame,
black sesame, squash, pumpkin, sunflower. Nuts maybe consumed less
often as they are higher in oil and more difficult to digest. Less oily nuts,
including almonds, peanuts and walnuts, may be lightly roasted, salted
and eaten as a snack occasionally. It is better to avoid more tropical nuts
(Brazil, cashew, etc.) and nut butters; sesame *tahini* may be used infrequently as an ingredient in cooking, and roasted sesame butter may be
used infrequently as a spread.

Snacks: It is better to eat balanced meals regularly and snack infrequently, as this establishes a stronger condition of the digestive system.
However, light snacks may be used occasionally, including: rice cakes,
popcorn and other puffed whole-grain products; lightly roasted or toasted
seeds or nuts (see above); roasted grains or beans; *sushi* (rice rolled with
vegetables or pickles and wrapped in *nori*) or rice balls; salads or pickles;
dried fruits.

Desserts: Sweet desserts may safely be enjoyed by persons in good
health up to three or four times per week; unsweetened cooked fruit
desserts or moderately sweetened grain or vegetable desserts are preferable.
Suitable ingredients include: sweet brown rice; sweet (hard) squashes or
pumpkin (other sweet vegetables such as parsnip or onion may also be
used); fresh or dried chestnuts; *azuki* beans; couscous; fresh or dried
northern or temperate climate fruits; nuts or seeds. *Suitable sweeteners*
(when needed) include: *amazake* (fermented sweet rice); rice syrup or
barley malt syrup; dried fruits (raisins, currants, dried apples, etc.) or
apple juice. *Suitable thickeners* for puddings and fillings include agar-agar
(*kanten*) and *kuzu* starch. In general, it is better to limit or avoid the use
of sweeteners on breakfast cereals or as a part of the main meal, as this
can interfere with good digestion. Also, the use of flour, granola toppings,
crusts and other processed grains in desserts is best kept to a minimum.

BEVERAGES: For sound digestion, it is best to avoid drinking during the meal. Also, since the macrobiotic way of eating has a somewhat higher water content in most dishes and is very low in animal proteins and fats (which can build to toxic levels in the kidneys), it is generally not necessary to drink excessive quantities. It is also better to avoid iced or cold drinks. Normally, a moderate serving of warm or hot beverage may follow a meal, with additional drinking during the day according to thirst. It is recommended to use unprocessed spring or deep-well water in preparation of all teas and beverages, as well as in cooking in general. *Beverages for daily or regular use* include: "*bancha*" twig tea, "*kukicha*" stem tea, roasted rice or roasted barley tea; boiled, spring or well water. *Beverages for occasional use* include: cereal grain coffee substitutes, roasted root beverages (dandelion, burdock or chicory "coffees"), *kombu* tea, *umeboshi* tea, *Mu* tea, or other non-aromatic, non-stimulant teas. *Beverages for* fresh vegetable *infrequent use in small amounts* include: *nachi* green tea; green magma; juices; temperate climate fruit juices (apple juice or cider is preferable, especially heated); naturally processed, high quality beer or rice wine (*sake*).

COOKING SEASONINGS: In general, all seasonings may be used lightly, and not obscure the natural taste of the ingredients used. Natural unrefined seasalt, traditionally prepared and aged *shoyu* (soy sauce) and *miso*, and *umeboshi* (dried pickled salt plum) may all be used mildly in cooking.

High quality, mechanically-expelled oils may be used up to two or three times per week in sautéing or frying (preferably just brushing the pan with an oil brush), and more infrequently for deep-frying or in dressings.

Suitable varieties include: sesame, dark or roasted sesame, squash or pumpkin, corn and mustard seed oil; sunflower, safflower, soy and olive oil may be used more infrequently, while peanut, coconut, palm and other heavier oils may be avoided.

Additional seasonings may be used in moderation to supply various tastes, including a sour taste (rice or other grain vinegar or *umeboshi* vinegar, naturally prepared sauerkraut or its juice), a pungent taste (fresh gingerroot, grated raw *daikon* or radish, chopped scallion or naturally prepared horseradish), or sweet taste (naturally prepared *mirin* sweet rice cooking wine, rice or barley malt syrup.)

TABLE CONDIMENTS: A variety of condiments may be used sparingly but regularly to impart additional nutrients and added flavor to various dishes. These include: baked sea vegetable powder, sea vegetable powder with crushed seeds, *gomashio* (finely ground seasalt mixed with crushed sesame seeds), ground *shiso* leaves, *umeboshi* plum, *tekka* (a traditional salted root vegetable powder), *shio kombu* (*kombu* stewed with *shoyu*) or *shio nori*, flakes, and others.

A small volume of naturally pickled vegetables can also be used regularly to accompany a meal. Macrobiotic pickles are prepared from a variety of vegetables, particularly *daikon* and other roots, broccoli, cauliflower and other ground vegetables, and more fibrous leafy vegetables such as kale or *daikon* greens, aged in salt or a salt, *shoyu* or *umeboshi* brine or other salt preparation, for from several hours to over a year.

Fresh vegetables garnishes, such as finely chopped scallions, parsley or watercress, may also be used in moderation to enhance the appearance and flavor of various dishes. Grated *daikon*, ginger or horseradish, usually seasoned with a little *shoyu*, are especially helpful for digestion of seafood, *mochi*, fried or deep-fried foods, or other slightly richer or heavier dishes.

Fig. 16.   Foods to be avoided for the betterment of health.

Animal Products:
Red meat (beef, lamb, pork)
Poultry
Wild Game
Eggs

Dairy Foods:
Milk (skim milk, buttermilk, etc.)
Butter
Cheese
Yogurt
Kefir
Ice cream
Cream (sour cream, whipped cream, etc.)

Fish:
Red meat or blueskinned fish, such as
   Tuna
Salmon
Swordfish
   Bluefish

Processed Foods:
Instant foods
Canned foods
Frozen foods
Refined (white) flour and its products
Polished (white) rice
Foods processed with:
   Chemicals
   Additives
   Preservatives
   Stabilizers
   Emulsifiers
   Artificial colorings, flavorings
Sprayed, dyed foods

Stimulants:
Spices (cayenne, curry, etc.)
Herbs
Vinegar (except natural grain vinegars)
Coffee
Commercial and dyed teas
Stimulating or aromatic teas (mint, rose hips, etc.)
Ginseng

Sweeteners:
Sugar (white, raw, brown, turbinado)
Honey
Molasses
Corn syrup
Date sugar
Fructose
Maple Syrup
Carob
Saccharine, xylitol and other artificial sweeteners

Fruits:
Tropical and sub-tropical fruits:

bananas	figs
grapefruits	prunes
mangoes	coconut
oranges	pineapple
papayas	kiwi
avocado	

Fats:
Lard or shortening
Margarine
Processed vegetable oils

Nuts:
Brazil
Cashew
Pistachio
Hazel

Beverages:
Artificial beverages, such as: soda, fruit punch, colas, etc.
Alcoholic beverages

The Way of Cooking

The way in which food is prepared has a powerful effect on its nutritional and other properties, and has a direct impact on health. In general, the kitchen should be kept clean, uncluttered and orderly, so that the cook's full attention can be given to proper cooking. Techniques such as stirring, mixing and vegetable cutting may be carried out with calm and orderly motions, and vegetables may be cut or chopped so that each piece is uniform, to ensure even and uniform cooking for each piece. It is preferable for dishes to be prepared fresh daily; leftovers can usually be stored at room temperature and lightly steamed or reheated when eaten. Refrigeration of leftovers may generally be avoided unless necessary, such as in very hot weather.

The use of longer cooking times, more salt and salt seasonings and pressure generally create dishes with a more yang effect, while the use of shorter cooking times, more water and other seasonings such as oil, vinegar or spicey tastes, and less pressure generally produce more yin effects. These two types of effects can be varied, and may be used to balance variations in climate, season and personal need. (For more information on this aspect of cooking, please refer to the *companion volume*.)

The type of cookware and stove used also affect the quality of the dishes themselves. It is preferable to use cookware made of traditional materials, such as cast iron, crockware, stoneware, stainless steel, enamel clad steel or iron, glassware, and others. Aluminum, teflon coated and other more artificial types of cookware may be avoided. Cooking over gas, wood or coal is preferable to the use of electric stoves, and microwave cooking is best avoided altogether.

The proper way of cooking is so important that the reader is strongly urged to attend qualified courses in macrobiotic cooking and to study independently with macrobiotic cookbooks.

The Way of Eating

In addition to the selection and preparation of the best ingredients, the way of eating itself has a strong impact on health. In general, upsetting, noisy or chaotic circumstances tend to disrupt digestion, and can contribute to a worsening health condition. Please try to eat only when calm, relaxed and unhurried; also, it is best to eat only when hungry.

Proper chewing is also essential for thorough digestion; each mouthful of food can be chewed at least thirty to fifty times, or until it is in liquid form and thoroughly mixed with saliva. Please try to avoid sleeping for three hours after eating, as this causes stagnation and weakness in the intestines.

When soup is part of the meal, it may be consumed as the first dish. Among various side dishes, the more yang, saltier or heavier dishes may be eaten earlier in the meal, with lighter dishes such as salads eaten toward the end of the meal; whole-grain dishes may be eaten throughout the meal. A warm or hot beverage may conclude the meal, or be followed by a reasonable portion of dessert if included. Eating foods too far out of this general order can also cause digestion to be disrupted.

Before and after each meal, it is a helpful practice to express your gratitude and appreciation verbally or silently to nature, the universe or God who created the food, and to reflect on the health and happiness it is dedicated to achieving. This acknowledgment may take the form of grace, prayer, song, chanting, a moment of silence or other traditional forms. To deepen your appreciation of the existence and significance of nature and its foods, you may also briefly express your thanks to parents, grandparents and ancestors who nourished us and whose dream we embody, to the vegetables or animals who gave their lives to nourish ours, and to the farmers, shopkeepers, cooks and other participants who contributed their energies in making the food available.

Dietary Adjustments for Diabetes and Hypoglycemia ——

When aiming to relieve a particular disorder, it is often helpful to adjust or modify the standard macrobiotic dietary approach. These modifications may generally be followed for an initial period of two to three months. As you begin to experience improvements, you may formally relax these adjustments and move towards the more general standard approach. All the suggestions below, therefore, are meant to be followed for an initial period of two to three months, and best under the guidance of an experienced macrobiotic counselor and/or appropriate medical professional.

Since both disorders reflect an imbalance in the level of blood glucose and in the body in general, the goal of cooking for both problems is to establish a consistent, balanced equilibrium. It is therefore important that individual dishes and menus as a whole not be one-sided—overly yin or overly yang—but reflect a harmonious balance of both energies at all times. Also, the way of eating and pattern of meals should be regular, consistent and orderly. For example, it is best to avoid periods of long fasting alternating with overly frequent eating or overeating.

Foods high in complex carbohydrate are especially helpful in establishing a smooth glucose metabolism; therefore, it is particularly important to include whole grains as at least one half of each meal. Grains and vegetables with a sweeter taste when well-cooked are especially helpful—these include: short grain brown rice, sweet brown rice and millet; hard squashes, pumpkin and Hokkaido pumpkin, onions, carrots, turnips, rutabagas, parsnips, green cabbage, *daikon*, leek, cauliflower. Other foods that are especially helpful include smaller beans (*azuki* and lentil) and more yang seeds (sesame and pumpkin). The sweetness of fruits and concentrated sweeteners or the use of refined or processed grains and grain products are generally not helpful as a regular source of carbohydrate.

Since the two disorders are different in nature and cause, the approach to both should also differ slightly. The guiding purpose in cooking for diabetes is generally to foster strength, endurance and a focusing or concentration of inner energy. Accordingly, a somewhat greater emphasis may be put on heartier, more well-cooked foods, with somewhat less emphasis on very light styles. Cooking for hypoglycemia, on the other hand, would aim more to dissolve stagnation and liberate blocked energies. Dishes may overall have a somewhat lighter, more refreshing appearance, with less emphasis on more yang preparations. Particular care can be taken to avoid dishes of an overly heavy, colorless or overcooked nature.

In both cases, the central issue is to avoid extremes and to recover stability, harmony and balance. The cook can take care to avoid sloppy, chaotic combinations of ingredients, overly repetitive menus or vague, "one-pot" styles of cooking. Each ingredient should be distinct, with each meal artistically and aesthetically harmonized as well as nutritionally balanced. With practice and good instruction, this ability can soon become a matter of common sense, and need not be a painstakingly complex effort.

For Diabetes	For Hypoglycemia

WHOLE GRAINS

General style: slightly more dry, chewier; pressure-cooking is preferred.

Emphasize: short grain brown rice, millet, sweet brown rice; occasionally using buckwheat.

Limit or avoid: corn and corn meal, flour or processed grains (may use macrobiotic quality whole-grain bread, *seitan*).

General style: may be slightly softer, more often using grain soups or creams; may be pressure-cooked and boiled.

Emphasize: short and medium grain brown rice, millet, sweet brown rice; barley and pearl barley.

Limit or avoid: buckwheat, all flour products; may occasionally use bulgur, cracked wheat, cracked rye.

SOUPS

Limit volume to one or two small cups per day; seasoning with *miso* or *tamari* may be slightly stronger. May often use *mochi* in soup.

May use larger volume of soups more often: seasoning with *miso* or *tamari* should be very light. May occasionally use *shiitake* mushroom.

VEGETABLES

In both cases, a small dish of hard squash, *azuki* beans and *kombu*, well cooked and seasoned with *tamari* soy sauce (more lightly seasoned for hypoglycemia, more strongly seasoned in the case of diabetes), may be eaten often or daily. When hard squashes are out of season, sweet tasting roots such as turnip or carrot may be substituted. Also, any round compact vegetables with a sweet taste may be used often or daily, including cabbage, onion, hard squash, rutabaga, turnip, and others.

General style: more long-time dishes (10–45 minutes); simpler, heartier dishes; slightly stronger seasoning with seasalt, *miso*, *shoyu* or *umeboshi*.

Emphasize: roots, hard squashes and all vegetables with a sweet taste (when cooked), leafy vegetables with a more complex leaf structure (kale, watercress, etc.)

Limit or avoid: vegetables listed as "occasional"—mushrooms, celery, lettuce, etc. (see p. 97)

General style: more medium- and short-time cooking (3–15 minutes); greater variety, lighter dishes; very light seasoning with seasalt, *miso*, *shoyu*, and *umeboshi*; more often boiled, pressed or raw salads.

Emphasize: hard squashes and all vegetables with a sweet taste (when cooked), all leafy vegetables; may use those vegetables listed as "occasional." (see p. 97)

BEANS

Use only: *azuki* and green lentil for the initial period, preferably cooked together with *kombu* and hard squash or other sweet vegetables; may use dried *tofu*, particularly cooked with sea vegetables; all seasoning may be slightly stronger.

Emphasize: *azuki*, green lentil and chickpea, especially cooked with sweet vegetables and *kombu*; may also use *tofu* (fresh or dried), *natto*, *tempeh*. All seasoning with seasalt, *miso* or *shoyu* should be lighter. May also garnish lightly with finely chopped scallion, celery leaves, or rice vinegar.

SEA VEGETABLES

Especially emphasize: *kombu*, *arame* and *hijiki*. A side dish of *arame* or *hijiki*, cooked with roots or sweet vegetables and seasoned with *shoyu* and several drops of oil, may be eaten 2–3 times per week.

Especially emphasize: *kombu*, *arame*, *wakame* and *nori*. A side dish of *arame*, cooked with sweet tasting vegetables and seasoned lightly with *shoyu* and several drops of brown rice vinegar, may be eaten 2–3 times per week.

SEEDS, NUTS, SNACKS

Use only sesame, black sesame and pumpkin seeds, lightly toasted and salted with seasalt or *shoyu*. A small volume of roasted peanuts or almonds may also be used regularly as a snack; tropical nuts should be avoided. Rice cakes and puffed whole grains may also be used.

Sesame, black sesame, pumpkin and sunflower seeds may be used either as ingredients in cooking or as a snack; however, it is best to avoid the excessive use of roasted, baked or dry-puffed foods. Nuts may generally be limited or avoided, with the exception of chestnuts.

SEAFOODS

If desired or needed for strength, a small volume of fresh white-meat fish may be used up to several times per week. All fish dishes may be served together with a small side dish of grated raw *daikon* and *shoyu*, natural horse-radish, finely chopped onion or scallion.

Fish and seafood are generally to be limited or avoided. If desired, a small volume of white-meat fish may be added to a lightly seasoned *miso* or *shoyu* soup to satisfy the craving for animal foods.

DESSERTS

In general, the sweetness of well-cooked, well-chewed grains and carbohydrate-rich vegetables should be emphasized as a regular part of meals. In addition, a lightly sweetened dessert may be eaten two to three times per week, as desired.

Emphasize: desserts prepared from sweet brown rice, hard squashes and other sweeter vegetables, *azuki* beans, chestnuts; more occasionally, you may use *amazake*, rice malt or barley malt syrup as sweeteners; and more infrequently, a small volume of dried or fresh cooked temperate climate fruit may be eaten, such as cooked apple with *kuzu*. It is generally better to avoid using very sweet dried fruits, fruit juices or sweet vegetable juices (e.g., carrot juice); however, these may occasionally be used if necessary, for example, to help recover from a hypoglycemic episode.

SEASONINGS FOR COOKING

A slightly saltier taste may be achieved with seasalt, *miso*, *shoyu* and *umeboshi*. However, as overuse of salt may lead to excessive thirst, all such seasonings may be moderate, and may need to be regularly adjusted as your individual needs change.

A small amount of oil may be used for sautéing or frying regularly or daily; high-quality, mechanically expelled sesame or dark (roasted) sesame oil is best for this purpose.

Fresh ginger, grated *daikon*, brown rice vinegar and *umeboshi* vinegar may be used very moderately. *Mirin* (sweet rice cooking wine), herbs, garlic, fruit vinegars and other seasonings may be avoided.

Seasalt, *miso*, *shoyu* and *umeboshi* should all be used more sparingly for a very mild taste; a small strip of *kombu* may be used in place of salt seasoning in some dishes.

The use of vegetable oils may generally be avoided until the hypoglycemic condition has improved.

Gingerroot, fresh *daikon*, rice vinegar and other macrobiotic quality seasonings may be used moderately. Garlic, herbs and other stronger seasonings may be avoided.

BEVERAGES

For daily or regular use: *bancha* twig and *bancha* stem teas, roasted rice or roasted barley teas. *For occasional use*: cereal grain or roasted root coffees, *kombu* tea, *umeboshi* tea, *Mu* tea.

In general, consumption of all beverages and liquids (including soups) may be very moderate.

For daily or regular use: *bancha* twig or *bancha* stem teas, roasted rice and roasted barley teas, spring or deep-well water. *For occasional use*: cereal grain or roasted root coffees, *kombu* tea.

Avoid: fruit juices, sweet vegetable juices, green tea, black teas and all stimulant or aromatic beverages, alcoholic beverages.

108

TABLE CONDIMENTS

For daily or regular use: *goma-shio*, made with a proportion of 12–14:1 (sesame seeds to seasalt) —it is best to use only homemade quality *gomashio*; baked and ground *kombu* or *wakame* powders; sea vegetable powders ground with crushed sesame or pumpkin seeds; *nori*, *umeboshi* plum.

For occasional use: *tekka*, *shio kombu*, *chirimen iriko* (dried tiny whole fish) powder.

Preferable pickles include those prepared from cabbage, kale and other more fibrous leaves, *daikon* and other roots, pickled for a minimum of several days in sea-salt brine, rice bran and seasalt or seasalt alone. Vegetables pickled for a minimum of three months such as *takuan* (long-term *daikon* pickles in rice bran and seasalt) or *miso* pickles are especially helpful.

For daily or regular use: *goma-shio*, with a proportion of about 16:1, preferably homemade; sea vegetable powders; sea vegetable powders ground with crushed seeds; *nori* or green *nori* flakes; *umeboshi* plum.

For occasional use: *shio nori*, rice vinegar, *shiso* leaves.

All macrobiotic quality pickles may be used, including quick-term pickles, naturally prepared sauerkraut, and others; however, pickles with an overly salty taste may be avoided.

Special Needs

It should be emphasized that every person is unique and has individual needs, and because of this it is strongly advisable to work together with a qualified macrobiotic advisor as well as the appropriate health professional when seeking to alleviate health problems. The suggestions given below are not meant to be followed as a prescription, but serve to illustrate some typical approaches that have traditionally been used in conjunction with the general macrobiotic guidelines given above. In the discussion below, all terms and recipes marked with an asterisk (*) are explained in more detail in the companion volume from the *Macrobiotic Food and Cooking Series*.

1. Digestive Problems. Make sure to maintain a calm, orderly way of eating, and especially emphasize chewing each bite thoroughly, one hundred times or more. Difficulties with digestion often disappear shortly after beginning a macrobiotic way of eating, without any special attention. However, for very weak digestion you may also take one small cup of *ume-sho-kuzu** each day for up to ten days. For stagnated bowel functions you may apply a hot ginger compress* over the abdomen, once each day for several days. Also, any stiff, painful or hardened areas may be deeply massaged each day, particularly in the shoulders, calves, buttocks and soles of the feet. Vigorous daily walks can also help strengthen absorption and digestion.

2. Eye Problems. Wash the eyes with warm *bancha* twig tea with a very small pinch of seasalt added to cleanse the eyes and help reduce irritation. For serious problems such as glaucoma, cataracts or retinitis, you may do this simple cleansing several times per day. In addition, you may use several drops of heated sesame oil*, first straining it through a cheesecloth, applied with an eyedropper.

3. Fatigue. For temporary fatigue you may drink a cup of *tamari-bancha** or *miso soup**; deep massage in the center of each palm can also help to rejuvenate your energy. If fatigue persists for several weeks after beginning to eat macrobiotically, check whether your application of the general guidelines may be too narrow or rigid. For example, your menus may be too monotonous or repetitive, or you may lack lightly or freshly cooked dishes. It may also be helpful to include a little more fish*, *mochi** or other slightly richer foods in your diet until you feel stronger.

4. Fat Accumulation. Even in thin persons, the accumulation of stagnated fats often prevents the glands and organs from functioning actively. To check for this condition, hold your hands together and bend your hands out at the fingers' base: you should be able to make a 90° angle (palms to fingers.) As another method of checking, lie on your back, with your knees up, and press with your fingers deep into your abdomen. If you feel pain or hardness, you likely have this condition of general fat accumulation. Again, adopting a general macrobiotic eating pattern will gradually dissolve and discharge this fat. To accelerate this process, in the case of hypoglycemia you may drink a cup of carrot-*daikon* tea* each day, for several weeks. In the case of diabetes, you may substitute a small cup of the broth from boiling a tablespoon of dried shredded *daikon**.

5. Headache. The headaches that often arise with hypoglycemia normally disappear as the hypoglycemia itself improves. However, a headache may temporarily reappear even when you are eating well, as a symptom of discharging previously stored toxins. If this headache arises more toward the front of the head, apply a cold, damp washcloth to the area; if more toward the rear, you may apply a warm washcloth. Massaging and pulling rhythmically out on the toes is also helpful, as is massaging any sensitive areas on the inside of the forearm.

6. *Infection.* Like headaches, low-grade infections often accompany hypoglycemia and may occasionally reappear, particularly if your diet has been temporarily compromised. With this condition, it is best to limit or avoid the use of oil, any flour products, fruits, animal foods and raw salads until the condition has been alleviated. You may use a cool plaster of mashed *tofu** and finely chopped, mashed raw greens (especially cabbage) to help reduce the fever over any infected area.

7. *Kidney Problems.* In the case of hypoglycemia the kidneys and adrenal glands often become stagnated with fats, or exhausted from constant over-stimulation (from sugar, excessive drinking, coffee, drugs or others), or both. This may produce: darkness or puffiness below and around the eyes, chronic fatigue, extreme sensitivity to cold or loud noises, or a pervasive feeling of fear, paranoia or inability to cope with stress. To help relieve this condition, it is best to carefully control your intake of salt and salt products, as well as liquids and sweets. Keep your feet warm in cold weather, and use a ginger compress* or hot water bottle on the mid-back to increase blood circulation to your kidneys and adrenals, two or three times per week. You may also drink a small cup of boiled *azuki* bean broth*, lightly seasoned with *tamari* or seasalt, several times per week, to strengthen these organs. (If you have been consuming too much salt, it is better to prepare this drink without any seasoning.)

In the case of the more severe kidney problems that may accompany diabetes, you may eat a small side dish of lotus root* or lotus seeds* boiled with *kombu* and seasoned with *tamari* soy sauce, several times per week, and use a hot ginger compress* over the kidney area daily, until you begin to experience some relief.

8. *Menstrual and Reproductive Problems. Amenorrhea*, the complete cessation of menstrual periods, is a common condition of hypoglycemic women; again, menstrual periods will usually resume within several months after beginning to eat macrobiotically, though this may in some cases take up to one year. To aid in dissolving and releasing stagnated animal fat and protein that can cause the reproductive system to become blocked, you

can use a *daikon* leaves hip bath,* followed by a douche made with *bancha* tea*; this can be used daily or regularly until the period resumes.

Diabetic men often suffer from a weakened sexual vitality. In this case, you should make sure to take vigorous daily exercise, and use some side dishes daily that include well-cooked root vegetables, such as carrot, burdock, dandelion root or *jinenjo* (mountain potato).

9. Skin Problems. Skin disorders are common complaints for those with either diabetes or hypoglycemia, as the skin is called upon to discharge accumulating waste products when the body's natural excretory mechanisms are blocked or weakened. If such a condition arises it is best to limit or avoid using oil, flour products, fruits or fruit juices, all animal foods, and raw salads until the condition improves. It is also especially important to avoid using any chemically produced cosmetics, as well as synthetic fabrics worn next to the skin. Wear cotton as much as possible, expose your skin to the fresh air daily, and for washing you may use a natural wash made by soaking a cheesecloth or cotton sack filled with rice bran* in warm water.

Overcoming Addictions and Cravings

To support the process of overcoming addictions or habitual reliance on various foods and substances, it is especially important to maintain a good range of variety in your selection of foods and styles of preparation. In making a transition to a more moderate way of eating, people often experience times when the taste, texture or stimulating qualities of previous foods suddenly become strongly attractive, leading to the desire to "binge" on some of those foods. Such occurrences may also give rise to a feeling of guilt, or a reinforcement of other negative feelings associated with the distinctions of "good" and "bad." However, we should strive to put aside these dualistic reactions, and use such occasions as opportunities for learning. Reflecting on such experiences, we often find that our macrobiotic practice has been overly restrictive, narrow or one-sided, for example, using only well-cooked dishes and none with a lighter, fresher taste. These experiences can be educational and lead to improved creativity in cooking. On the other hand, in the case of a true addiction it is important that such problems are offset before they arise, as it is better to completely avoid slipping back into use of the item in question.

If you experience cravings for specific foods, it is often helpful to consume moderate amounts of high-quality foods having a similar taste, texture, or other property of the food craved. The following chart provides some examples of how this principle can be applied.

Craving	Transitional Food	Ideal
Meat	fish, seafood	well-cooked *seitan*, *tempeh*, *tofu* beans
Eggs, dairy foods, fatty or greasy foods	fried or deep-fried grains, beans, bean products; nuts, nut butters, soy milk	soy products: *tempeh*, *tofu*, *natto*; roasted seeds
Tropical fruits & juices, artificial beverages, cold drinks	organic temperate-climate fruits, juices	organic temperate-climate fruits (dried or cooked) and juices in small volume and in season
Sugar, sweets	honey, maple syrup	cooked or dried fruits, natural grain sweeteners
Strong alcohol	high-quality beer, *sake* (rice wine) in small volume	fermented grain, bean and vegetables foods: *tempeh*, sauerkraut, fresh pickles, *amazake*, *miso*, etc.
Coffee, black tea, soft drinks, diet drinks	herb teas, green tea, mineral water	*bancha* twig tea, grain coffees, root coffees

In the case of alcoholism, it is particularly important to consume some fermented food daily, including *tempeh*, *miso* (used in seasonings and sauces as well as in soups), sauerkraut and other naturally tart-tasting pickles, *amazake*, or naturally-raising sourdough bread. In addition, be careful to include some fresh-tasting, lightly cooked vegetable dish or dishes each day. The overuse of salt and salt seasonings can easily lead to intensified cravings, and in the case of both alcoholism and all addictions or consistent cravings, salt use should be carefully controlled. If even a minimal amount of salty seasonings still seems to be too strong for your use, you may temporarily eliminate its use and substitute *kombu* or *wakame* powder for cooking and seasoning.

Medications

After adopting a macrobiotic lifestyle and way of eating, it is a common experience for various health conditions to improve to the point where is it possible to discontinue the use of some medications. However, the question of when, how gradually and whether at all it is advisable to discontinue medications is a highly individual issue, and is best approached with reasonable caution and in consultation with the appropriate medical professional.

As a general rule, a reliance on drugs or medications should be withdrawn gradually rather than all at once, in stages that follow the gradual change in health and permit a regular reassessment of dosages and their effects. Most prescription and non-prescription medications fall into one of three categories. *Supplements and miscellaneous aids* such as sleeping pills, sedatives, stimulants, pain killers, vitamin and mineral tablets, and others, can usually be discontinued fairly quickly, over a period of ten days to two months. Medicines that *affect or control bodily conditions* include blood pressure medications, diuretics, antibiotics, anticonvulsives, anti-inflammatory drugs such as cortisone, and others. As the condition in question improves, these can often be withdrawn gradually over a period of about one to four months.

The third category includes medications that *maintain or regulate vital bodily functions*, including hormone supplements or replacement and anti-diabetic oral drugs. Mechanical supports would also come under this category, including such devices and procedures as pacemakers, dialysis, insulin pumps and routine catherization. Naturally, treatments in this third category must be approached with the greatest caution, and generally take the longest time to withdraw. This may take anywhere from several months up to one or two years, and in cases where an organ or gland has been removed or has completely lost functioning ability, the supply of medications or hormones may need to be continued at some level for a lifetime.

In general, it is usually possible to discontinue using oral anti-diabetic drugs within a reasonably brief period. Diabetic patients undergoing routine insulin therapy commonly find that their level of insulin needs begins to change rapidly upon adopting a macrobiotic lifestyle, and the patient should carefully monitor himself and frequently adjust the dosage, preferably under medical supervision, to avoid unnecessarily overdosing. Whether or not an insulin-dependent diabetic patient can completely discontinue the use of insulin therapy depends on many factors, such as how long he or she has been relying on insulin injections, whether or not the pancreas is capable of some degree of regeneration, the severity of extremes in previous dietary patterns, and others.

It is fairly common for Type I diabetic patients to reach a certain point— when the insulin dosage has been reduced to anywhere from one-half to one-tenth of the original level—where improvement suddenly becomes much slower, and it becomes very difficult to reduce the dosage any further. Subsequently, he may even find his insulin needs slightly rising again, and continuing to fluctuate around this low threshold. At this time, the patient's overall condition is adjusting to its new metabolism, and may be discharging very deep, long-term accumulations of poor quality foods. Under these circumstances, it is especially important to continue eating within the general macrobiotic guidelines, and not slip into previous more chaotic eating habits.

At the same time, it is equally important to avoid being overly rigid, and to maintain a flexible approach within those guidelines. For example, though it may be better in terms of strengthening the pancreas to avoid eating any fruits or sweets, the person's overall system may have changed so substantially and discharged so much excess, that a slightly broader approach including some cooked fruit, sweet macrobiotic dessert dishes, salads or other dishes becomes appropriate. The same idea applies to those recovering from hypoglycemia: even before the hypoglycemic condition has completely disappeared, there may be times when a somewhat broader approach to macrobiotic eating seems appropriate. It is vitally important to exercise your own intuition in such circumstances, as there is no hard and fast rule of thumb that can be followed. As in all areas of life, the appropriate way to eat macrobiotically can never be reduced to set formulas or rigid rules, because each person is a unique, constantly changing manifestation of nature. Initially, as we follow written guidelines or principles learned through cooking classes or cookbooks, macrobiotic cooking and eating often appears to be a technique or science; but as our awareness of the dynamic nature of our health and our food grows, we gradually begin to realize that eating macrobiotically is truly an art.

6. Towards a Balanced Way of Life━━━━

In order to establish a firm foundation of natural health, it is essential that we recognize those factors that have originally led to our suffering or sickness, so we can seek to correct them. Hypoglycemia and diabetes are symptoms of a generally disorderly lifestyle, of which chaotic or excessive habits of eating and drinking are the central but not the only feature. When we reflect on the way of living that has resulted in an unbalanced metabolism, we can usually discover many areas in which our behavior has been chronically extreme or one-sided, or in some way cut off from the natural energies and rhythms of yin and yang that animate the world around us. Let us examine seven general areas where we can direct our attention towards creating a more harmonious, natural way of life.

1. Harmony in Daily Lifestyle Habits━━━━━━━

Every aspect of daily living has both yang and yin or active and passive aspects. For example, we naturally balance eating with fasting, more physical with more mental activities, and more active periods with more restive times. In seeking to establish a more harmonious metabolic pattern, it is also helpful to maintain a balanced regularity within these aspects of living as well. This would include the following suggestions:

- You may eat as often as you like, but it is better to leave the table feeling satisfied and not full. While suffering from blood sugar disorders (particularly hypoglycemia), it may be helpful to eat smaller meals up to six times per day, rather than larger meals less often. It is better to eat regularly, with a consistent meal pattern, than to alternate between eating a great deal on some days and more sporadically on others.
- Eat with good appetite and in a relaxed, unhurried manner, chewing each bite thoroughly until it becomes liquid in your mouth. Try to avoid drinking while you eat; drink comfortably, after or between meals, enough to satisfy your thirst.
- It is better to avoid lengthy, hot baths or showers as they can deplete your body of minerals and have a weakening effect. Bathe as needed, but preferably use brief baths or showers with a moderate temperature. If you feel fatigued after bathing, you may drink a small cup of hot *tamari*-bancha* to replenish your energy.
- To vitalize your blood and lymph circulation, scrub and massage

every part of your body with a hot, damp towel until the skin becomes red, each morning or night. At the least, scrub the arms, legs, hands and feet, including each finger and toe. In addition, some regular *shiatsu* or *Do-In* massage may help recover a vital and balanced metabolism.[1]

- Using hot compresses occasionally may help revitalize stagnated functions with increased blood circulation. In the case of hypoglycemia, you may apply a very hot, damp towel across the front of the abdomen, just under the rib cage (the region including the liver, gall bladder, spleen, stomach and pancreas); change the towel as it cools, continuing for about fifteen to twenty minutes. This can be done several times per week. In the case of diabetes, a hot ginger compress* applied over the pancreas region can be helpful in some cases, though it is often not necessary. For guidance in this it is best to seek the advice of an experienced macrobiotic counselor.

- Include some regular physical activity in your daily life, including activities such as scrubbing floors, cleaning windows, washing and cleaning your home, carpentry, gardening, and others. Some form of systematic exercise program may be very helpful, such as yoga, *Do-In* (self massage), martial arts, athletics, regular long walks, and others; in the case of diabetes, some slightly more strenuous physical activity may be particularly beneficial. Some regular deep breathing exercises can also help to increase the body's discharge of accumulated toxins, regulate the metabolism, and calm your mind. Sample exercises are provided in the companion volume.[2] Try to establish a regular schedule of exercise and adequate rest, rather than sporadically alternating periods of strenuous exercise with long sedentary periods.
- For the deepest and most restful sleep, and to help establish an even metabolism, it is best to retire before midnight and rise early in the morning. Please avoid eating for three hours before sleeping, and avoid drinking for about thirty minutes before sleeping.

2.   Harmony with the Natural Environment

In addition to the direct use of the fuel energies in food and drink, the body's functions rely constantly on the energies of air, heat, light and more subtle electromagnetic forces conducted to us by the sun, stars, atmosphere, soil, and plant world around us. In order to recover from illness and to maintain vital health, we can keep an active contact and exchange with these natural forces, and minimize the interfering and more chaotic energies caused by excessively artificial environments.

• Go outdoors often, lightly dressed when possible, and try to walk
  barefoot on the soil, grass or beach every day. Keep large green plants
  in your home to enrich and freshen the oxygen content of the air; and
  open your windows whenever you can to permit fresh air to circulate.

• All daily living materials should be as natural as possible, as synthetic
  fabrics and other materials can disrupt the energies you receive from
  the natural environment. Wear cotton clothing directly next to your
  skin, especially your undergarments, and avoid wearing synthetic,
  woolen or silk clothing that touches your skin. Excessive metallic
  jewelry or accessories on the fingers, neck or wrists are best kept
  to a minimum. Cotton sheets, towels, blankets and pillowcases, and
  incandescent lighting, natural wooden furnishings, or wool carpeting
  all contribute to a more natural environment.

• Avoid or minimize the use of electric appliances close to the body,
  including electric shavers, hair dryers, blankets, heating pads, tooth-
  brushes, etc. It is especially advisable to use a gas or wood stove for
  all cooking rather than electric or microwave devices. It is also
  preferable to use earthenware, glassware, cast iron or stainless steel
  cookware rather than aluminum, teflon coated or electric cooking
  pots.

• Television, particularly color television, exerts a draining influence on
  the body, as do all ionizing radiation devices such as computer display
  terminals, video games and X-ray machines. If you watch television,
  do so in moderation and from a reasonable distance, and keep your
  contact with all such devices to a minimum.

• To maintain the healthy functioning of your skin, which helps the
  excretory system in the regular discharge of toxins, avoid using
  chemically produced cosmetics and body care products; try to use
  those natural cosmetics made from vegetable sources only. For care
  of teeth, use natural toothpaste, seasalt, *dentie** or clay.

3. Harmony in Behavior and Expression ━━━━━━

Disorders in blood glucose metabolism are usually accompanied by some
extreme or unbalanced patterns of behavior. The accompanying figure,
for example, illustrates some common types of extreme expression, seen in
terms of their relatively more yin or more yang nature.

More Yang	More Yin
domineering	complacent
aggressive	defensive, negative
over-confident	under-confident
self-asserting	self-denying
overly concerned with the past	overly concerned with the future
denial of spiritual or philosophical affairs	denial of material or practical affairs
exclusion of others	dependency on others

It is best to avoid such extremes, and strive for a varied but more moderate, balanced pattern of behavior.

4.   Harmony in Mind and Emotions

Blood glucose disorders, and particularly hypoglycemia, are often associated with a wide range of emotional and psychological patterns of disharmony. In many cases, such chronic disharmonies can themselves also contribute to a worsening overall condition, and can therefore be considered "cause" as well as "effect." These problems will tend to correct themselves automatically over time, as you establish a more harmonious blood glucose level through proper diet and lifestyle practices.

At the same time, the decision to begin establishing a more balanced, health-supporting diet and lifestyle should include a resolve to adopt a more positive, optimistic outlook. Seek to live each day happily, without being preoccupied with your condition or dwelling on negative thoughts or emotions. If such negative feelings do arise, it is often helpful to realize that they are simply the result of an internal biochemical imbalance, and they will pass; this can help to dispel any unnecessary feelings of hopelessness.

The change from sickness to health, or from unhappiness to happiness, rarely proceeds in a straight line—you will probably experience transient periods of feeling worse, alternating with times of more clear-cut improvement when you feel much better. This is actually a naturally occurring cycle, and is an example of the universal rhythm of yin and yang which exists everywhere. During any more difficult periods, it is also helpful to read the personal accounts of those whose lives have changed through adopting macrobiotics, such as the experiences recounted in the next chapter. It is also helpful to renew and strengthen your contact with nature, and to keep up an active exchange with your family and friends, rather than isolating yourself.

The chart below illustrates some of the changes in mental state that are commonly experienced by people who adopt a macrobiotic way of life and diet.

irritation, anger, impatience	⟶ patience, amusement, humor
anxious, tense, "bottled up"	⟶ relaxed but purposeful, easily directed energies
complaining, critical, cynical	⟶ constructive energy, a sense of ability to positively change circumstances
depressed, isolated	⟶ an underlying, constantly joyful sense of continuity with nature and with other people
hopelessness, helplessness	⟶ confidence
apathy, lack of zest	⟶ self-motivation, energetic, easily inspired, a sense of wonder at the orderliness of nature
extreme swings of mood and energy	⟶ a more moderate, natural rhythm of more active and more restive mood and energy

5. Harmony in Relations with Family, Friends and Society

As your physical and personal sense of well-being grows, this naturally tends to extend out to your exchanges with those around you. Even in cases where one person eats macrobiotically and other family members or friends continue to eat and live in a way that may harm their health, a deeper sense of unity and harmony can be created by exercising a more peaceful and gracious expression. Helpful daily practices in this area would include:

- Greet everyone you meet happily and with appreciation.

- Initiate and maintain an active, regular correspondence with all family members, often expressing your gratitude.

- Enlarge your circle of friends and acquaintances, including people from all walks of life.

- Share your food with others often; food prepared in larger quantities is always more satisfying, and the act of sharing good food is a universal expression of human brotherhood and sisterhood.

● Put aside some time daily to make yourself quiet and peaceful, and offer your thanks to your ancestors, teachers and elders, and your dedication to help and suppprt those who will look to you for guidance. This may take the form of a simple meditation or prayer, or a simple daily dedication towards the furthering of human peace and happiness.

6.   Harmony through Daily Self-Reflection ───────

Our state of health is a reflection of our way of viewing ourselves. Sickness results not only from poor choices in daily food and drink, but also from a generally unhappy or distorted self-image. Living in the modern technological, fast-paced world, we may easily come to see ourselves as separate from the rest of the world, as lone beings fighting for survival against hostile surroundings.

By adopting a more universal, embracing perspective, we begin to see that we are not at all separate, but are manifestations of the natural world that has created us and constantly provides us with air, sunlight and nourishment. In taking responsibility for our own health, we can extend this view to all aspects of our lives; and we begin to realize that all the influences in our daily lives, even apparent failures, sickness or difficulties, are serving to support us and challenge us to strengthen our own capabilities. By appreciating the gift of life in all its dimensions, we increase our faith in the integrity of the universe, and life increasingly becomes a joyful and amusing adventure.

The practice of self-reflection involves using our higher consciousness to observe, review, examine and evaluate our thoughts and behavior, and to contemplate the larger order of nature or what we may call the law of God. Whenever we experience failings or difficulties, seeing ourselves and our lives in this larger perspective allows us to draw on the greatest resources both within and without. As a daily practice to develop and deepen this sort of awareness, self-reflection may take the form of quiet prayer or meditation, as described in the section above. Questions we might ask and areas wherein we might seek guidance may include the following:

1.   Did I eat today in harmony with my environment, my history and my purpose in life?

2. Did I think of my parents, relatives, friends, teachers and elders with love and respect?
3. Did I happily greet everyone I met today and express an interest in their lives?
4. Did I contemplate the sky, trees, plants and stars, and marvel at the wonders of nature?
5. Did I contemplate the works of art, culture, industry, and human ingenuity and endeavor, and marvel at the aspirations of human society?
6. Did I thank everyone and appreciate everything I experienced today?
7. Did I carry out my activities today with faith and commitment, and thereby contribute to the dream of a more peaceful world?

7. Harmony with Life Purpose

People respond in different ways to the changes brought about by the macrobiotic way of eating. Some people begin to experience improvements in health, even successfully recovering from major chronic illnesses, but feel no desire to carry this change into other areas of their lives. They may avoid sharing their experiences with others, preferring to keep their way of eating to themselves, and continue as much as possible with their previous activities and way of life. People in this category often stop eating macrobiotically after they have achieved some measure of improvement in health, and return to their previous eating habits, frequently with an eventual return of health problems.

Others have the opposite experience, and are so excited by their new-found state of well-being that they cannot help but share their discoveries openly and enthusiastically with all around them. These people usually find that the positive redirection felt in their health gradually permeates every aspect of their lives, as a more or less permanent transformation.

When we are first learning about the macrobiotic approach, we naturally tend to focus on the dietary aspect, and simply changing our eating habits is often enough to begin improving the way we feel. But to maintain this positive direction, we soon feel the need for deeper changes in the way we live. For example, we may begin to reflect more deeply on the direction of our professional careers—if you are eating macrobiotically and are an executive in a company that produces sugared foods, microwave ovens or components for nuclear armaments, it is only natural that a sense of conflict should arise. We often don't realize how deeply the implications of our eating habits reach until we have significantly changed the way we ourselves eat every day.

As we change the quality of our blood and body cells and our approach to health, nature and life itself, we gradually begin to experience that the whole of society is presently moving in a generally unhealthy, destructive direction; and we naturally seek to contribute positively toward the reorientation of this movement as an expression of our daily way of life.

When we closely observe the world around us, we can see that there are two major currents emerging in society today, which supercede all other distinctions such as capitalist versus communist, rich versus poor, old versus young or male versus female. The first current is characterized by more extreme behavior, moving towards increasingly artificial solutions to the various problems we face. Particularly in the field of health, we can see a rapidly growing trend towards the use of organ transplants and artificial organs, genetic manipulation and other aspects of what is now called "biotechnology." Rather than seeking to uncover the cause of our health problems through commonsense self-reflection, and implementing a course of prevention through returning to more moderate, natural patterns of behavior, this direction tends to ignore the cause of problems and cope temporarily with their outward symptoms through increasingly artificial means.

The second current is characterized by self-reflection: when problems arise, we look inward to search out what aspects of our own behavior have been out of harmony. Rather than continuing our own disruptive behavior and trying to change nature itself, we instead realize that nature is not at fault but is in fact our own source and origin; and we attempt to adapt ourselves to better conform with its laws. This needn't require that we abandon the ideal of progress, nor should we be afraid to apply our natural human ingenuity to the pursuit of technology. On the contrary, we can be free to enjoy tremendous technical achievements, as long as these achievements do not disrupt the natural harmony of the order of the universe.

	Degenerative	*Constructive*
Historical attitude	discarding traditions	adapting traditions
Approach to problems	blaming, seeking external cause	self-reflective, seeking internal cause
Method of solution	technological, artificial	organic, natural
Characteristic action	replace defective part	reorient disharmonious whole
Outlook	analytical	comprehensive
Behavior	extreme, disruptive	moderate, harmonious
Blood glucose tendency	hyper- or hypoglycemia	normoglycemia

In over half a century's experience, we have been able to see the results of the artificial approach in the field of diabetes treatment. Though first heralded as the precursor of a new era for diabetics, the practice of supplying insulin through injection has in fact done nothing to halt the increase of the disease, nor to abate its debilitating complications. We may project that the same type of ultimate failure will hold true for all highly artificial methods, such as in vitro-fertilization for impaired fertility, genetic engineering for a weakened agriculture, or robotics for a faltering global economy. In all areas of human experience, we need to turn inward to reflect on where we have abandoned commonsense values and disrupted the natural order, in order to find harmonious solutions to our multiple ills and realize our universal dreams of planetary health, happiness, peace and freedom.

The decision to eat macrobiotically therefore carries with it a broad meaning in today's troubled world. While it is a positive step towards taking responsibility for redirecting our own health and life, it is at the same time an action with planetary implications, an individual's "consumer vote" for a global reorientation towards a more moderate, healthier and more peaceful way of life.

---

[1] For a discussion of these practices, please refer to the author's *The Book of Do-In* and *Barefoot Shiatsu* by Shizuko Yamamoto, listed in the bibliography.
[2] Please refer to the *Book of Do-In* for an extensive treatment of breathing and exercise programs.

7. Personal Experiences ━━━━━━━━━━

Diabetes and Kidney Failure: Aron Weinstock ━━━━━

My name is Aron Weinstock. I was born on December 26, 1945 in Czechoslovakia, and lived in Antwerp, Belgium and Buenos Aires, Argentina until I settled in the United States in 1951. I now live in the Village of Kiryas Joel, in Monroe, New York, with my wife and ten children. I have been an accountant for 19 years.

In 1967 my health first began to deteriorate, with an elevated blood glucose level, borderline elevated blood pressure, and signs of kidney function problems. I began a series of visits to all kinds of specialists, including the head nephrologist at Mt. Sinai Hospital in New York. I received a diagnosis of partial renal failure, but none of the doctors I visited were sure exactly what was happening, nor could they offer any relief. An ultra-sound picture revealed that the nephrons, particularly in the left kidney, were shrunken so that I had, in that kidney, approximately 60 percent kidney function. I was advised there was nothing medically that could be done. With a diagnosis of diabetes in 1968 I began taking insulin intravenously, and my condition unfortunately continued to gradually worsen.

Then, although I was hoping very much this wouldn't happen, I eventually had to go onto dialysis, several years ago. Rather than hemodialysis, in which the blood is filtered through a dialysis machine during visits to the hospital, I chose the option of peritoneal dialysis, in which a catheter is surgically inserted into the peritoneum, and a dextrose solution is periodically injected into the peritoneal cavity, left for a while to clean out the toxins that accumulate due to the poor kidney function, and then is let out again. I went onto a routine of four visits per week, during which I would stay overnight at the hospital for eight hours of dialysis.

At this point, generally speaking, I felt I had no real life in me, no real desire to do anything, no concentration—I just maintained my day to day activities. Then I went to the New England Deaconness Hospital to be trained in home dialysis. They gave me a machine which I kept at home, and would hook myself up to this machine four times per week and go through the eight hours of dialysis while I slept. After about six or seven months, I found the fact that I was still tied to a machine to be a tremendous nuisance; I couldn't go away for any longer than a day or two. So I learned of another possibility: C.A.P.D., or Continuous Ambulatory Peritoneal Dialysis. This consists of a bag containing two liters of dialysis fluid, which is hung up on a pole and sends the fluid into the peritoneal cavity through the catheter by the power of gravity. This bag is changed every four hours. The advantage of this is that it is fully portable; but I began to have recurrent kidney infections, and eventually was put into the hospital for several months because they had to change the catheter.

While I was in the hospital, my wife gave me a copy of one of Mr. Kushi's book *Cancer and Heart Disease.* I read the book cover to cover, and noticed that a number of the case histories made reference to kidney problems; so while in the hospital I called the East West Foundation and made an appointment to see Mr. Edward Esko. As soon as I was discharged I went straight to Boston with my wife, and saw Mr. Esko, who gave me recommendations which I began to follow immediately and have continued to follow, with revisions and modifications in the meantime, ever since.

When I first began the diet, I didn't believe in it very strongly. The doctors had said it was virtually impossible for anyone to ever get off of this dialysis routine. However, within only several days I began to notice some remarkable changes. Ordinarily, for example, I would gain about five pounds of water accumulation over a weekend (without dialysis), which would come off again only when I would go through another night of dialysis. Yet, after my first weekend of macrobiotics, and without any dialysis at all, I actually lost six pounds. I also noticed that I felt more alert, began to require less sleep, and began to have very regular bowel movements. I continued to stay off dialysis; and the improvement in my diabetes allowed me to drastically reduce my insulin.

Nine weeks later I was visiting one of my doctors who had just run a a blood analysis. He said that I might be able to reduce the amount of dialysis that I was doing, because my blood profiles were excellent, showing practically normal levels. I told him he better sit down for this: "I haven't been on dialysis, not even once, for the past nine weeks." He couldn't believe it! Later, three months after I had begun macrobiotics and had stopped dialysis, one of my doctors clearly stated that this was "a miracle": neither he nor any of his colleagues could understand how it could be possible that I would be showing normal kidney function in my blood tests. At the same time, I had decreased my insulin dosage from about 45 units daily to 6 units daily.

Since that time I have continued to work with my doctors and to see Mr. Kushi, Mr. Esko and other macrobiotic counselors to have my condition monitored and my diet adjusted when necessary. My improvement has not been perfect—at one point when I had not been eating properly for my condition, I even had to take several dialysis treatments again—but the miracle continues; and I thank God I have finally found a way to reverse my previous direction of deterioration towards the opposite direction, of ever improving health and vitality.

Diabetes: Larry Bogoslaw

I was diagnosed as having Type I diabetes in October 1972 at the age of eight. I had always liked sweets, and I had a problem with bedwetting since I was four, but had not had any real problems with my health. I remember the night of my cousin's Bar Mitzvah: I hadn't eaten all day, and I was so hungry by the end of the evening that I binged on as much cake as I could eat. The next morning I threw up and began to feel really fatigued. My mother took me to a pediatrician, and the diagnosis was diabetes; I was put on one shot of insulin per day.

In the first few years I recall always being angry—I had cut sugar out of my diet, but I was still eating plenty of meat—and I lacked the will power to stay on the structured diet plan I was given. By the time I was eleven another doctor put me on two shots a day in an effort to better control my blood sugar, since I wasn't eating as carefully as I was supposed to. From the start, I was always a very undisciplined eater and drinker, and very poor at following any doctor's instructions; in fact, developing the ability to be orderly and disciplined in my approach to taking care of myself has been one of the biggest changes I have experienced now in my year of practicing macrobiotics.

In 1980 my father discovered macrobiotics in Philadelphia through the East West Foundation. Although my father began eating macrobiotically right away, I didn't begin until I came to Boston in June of 1983, where I had my first macrobiotic consultation and was given a completely different way to eat. At this time I was taking 65 units of insulin a day. Dr. Marc Van Cauwenberghe, the consultant I saw, told me I could possibly be taking as little as five or ten units of insulin by the end of the summer, and I was sure he was crazy! After about ten days of eating this way, I had been able to decrease my insulin dosage, dropping by ten percent increments, from 65 units to 46 units. By June 20th it was down to 35 or 40 units, and by some time in July it went down to 30. Early in August a new and more experienced macrobiotic cook moved into the apartment where my father and I were staying, and after a short period of eating her cooking, my insulin suddenly took another leap downwards. Now the daily insulin dosage is down to about 15 units.

In addition to the decrease in my insulin intake, I soon noticed a number of other changes. My acne diminished to a few small, dull bumps on my cheeks, and my complexion was brighter; my shoulders were suddenly straighter, and my energy calm and consistent from 8 A.M. to midnight. As the weeks became months these changes were accentuated, and more deep-seated transformations became apparent as well. Most importantly, it became clear that one old, deeply ingrained assumption of mine was no longer true. This was the assumption that I would not live past the age of thirty-five. With the constant feeling of my vitality ebbing away, every year and every month, this reality had become a constant background in my awareness and approach to life—and now this is gone. My vitality is ever increasing, and I am enjoying every minute of it, since I know that all my dreams, all my potential will be realized. If I can change this much in a year, anybody else can change even more so!

Diabetes: Susan Grindell

I was never a big sugar eater, because my mother was pretty strict about controlling the quality of what her kids ate. For example, she let us have soft drinks only once a week (on "popcorn night"). But we really ate a lot of dairy food, more than anything else. Also, by the time I was in high school I had already begun to have experiences with drugs among my friends—somehow I had the idea that taking drugs (marijuana) was much safer than alcohol, and I experimented with just about everything that was around at that time.

When I was 14 I had my first experience with LSD; true to my extreme nature, shortly after taking the first one I was enjoying myself so much that I took another. I don't know how much I can really blame on this experience, but it must have touched things off: right away I felt a pain radiating from my middle around my left side, and within a week I began to show some of the classic symptoms of Juvenile Onset diabetes. My appetite doubled, and my thirst became absolutely unquenchable; I was going to urinate every half hour. I mentioned this to a friend's mother one day and she commented, "Hm, that sounds an awful lot like diabetes." I went to my parents and said, "What can you tell me about diabetes?" My father laughed and said, "Oh, you don't have to worry about that, there's no chance you'll have that problem." Maybe he thought that because there was no history of diabetes in my family at all (which for me shoots a hole in the hereditary theory); but finally I said, "Okay, something's really wrong here, I've got to get to a doctor," and they took me.

Well, my blood sugar was over 800! The doctor said, "I honestly don't know how you're walking around." (Unlike a lot of diabetics I've met, I don't seem to have much trouble with highs in my sugar, but have always had the worst symptoms and biggest problems with hypoglycemic episodes.) They put me on a 1,200 calorie diet and slapped me in the hospital for 2 weeks, and when I got out I'd learned how to inject about 55–60 units of

Lente [slow-acting] insulin once a day. Later on they wanted me to go to two shots a day, but I refused. I'm a very extreme person, and I've always tended to ignore others' advice and go my own way. In fact, I really have no sense of discipline, and never had—it's no wonder I'm diabetic.

Putting me on insulin didn't slow me down. Like other diabetics I've met, I used insulin as a crutch, varying my dose to support my extreme behavior. College was a wild time for me. Though I was never much for sugar, alcohol became my binge; at one point I started to even get worried about becoming an alcoholic. During this time I had quite a few hypoglycemic episodes, and got myself into pretty serious trouble more than once. On one occasion I felt I was losing touch with reality and began to feel as if I were two people. My friends were there desperately spreading honey on bread and trying to get it down my throat while struggling to get me to go to the hospital (with no help from me!) Once I did get there, I had a blood sugar level of 40, and they suspected it had gotten as low as 20.

I left college, after 2 years, bought a house, and got a job. I knew about macrobiotics vaguely as early as 1976 or '77, but I didn't really start to dabble with it until 1980. First I became a vegetarian (still using dairy foods), and this change alone allowed me to drop ten units of insulin a day. After I began eating somewhat macrobiotically I dropped another ten units, down to 40 per day. But I didn't get really serious about macrobiotics until I moved to Boston in January of 1983, when I moved into a study house and started attending classes at the Kushi Institute. Since that time, I've resisted the urge to try and cut down drastically, and cutting out two units at a time, I've been able to drop very comfortably down to about 33 units per day—no small achievement, since I was on almost twice that for ten years.

But more dramatic for me than numbers is the way I feel. When I was first here in Boston I would wake up having a hypoglycemic episode, and within five minutes I'd be shaking. I'd know that if I didn't get some apple juice fast, I'd be in trouble. Now when I wake up with that feeling I can say, "Oh, I've got to correct this today." I can roll over and get a few more hours of sleep, or get up and go about my business for a while, and eventually go downstairs to fix a little sweet squash, or sometimes I may need a little cooked fruit. No more desperate dashes to the kitchen! For the first time in my life, I can really say that I'm not so extreme, and I'm in control of myself.

And more than control, I'm getting a true understanding of what's going on in my body. A friend recently pointed out that I might be eating a little too much salt; and just cutting down my salt use a tiny bit had me feeling much lighter and more balanced within a few weeks. I used to be incredibly dull at times, and couldn't feel what was going on; now I am aware of every little detail, and have become so much more sensitive. Of course, I hope to keep reducing the amount of insulin I need, and my health still has a long way to go. But at this point, with what I've learned from macrobiotics and the control and understanding it's given me, I consider myself a happier, luckier and, yes, healthier person than most!

Hypoglycemia: Faye Dresner

My struggle with hypoglycemia first became noticeable in high school. At that time I was using marijuana pretty heavily, and gradually I had become depressed—so depressed that someone just walking over and saying, "Hi, how are you?" would make me feel like sobbing! I had my happy times, but my mood was so volatile and extreme that I would plummet back into a profound feeling of despair. I never contemplated suicide, yet many times I thought I was "going crazy" as I felt so out of control, and I always had a feeling of wanting to escape. I felt very isolated, even paranoic at times, although it's ironic that my friends didn't see me as being unusually anti-social or withdrawn—it was really just my own negative perception of myself. Fortunately, I was always athletically inclined, and I think it was regular exercise that saved me from really losing my mind.

As bad as things were in high school, I was still somewhat dulled to how I was feeling, partially because of all the marijuana. It was when I got to college that I started to become a more aware, feeling person, which in some ways made things worse because I began to realize just how bad I felt! I was convinced after a while that my unhappiness was a result of some childhood emotional traumas and as a result went through two years of therapy—at one point I had psychotherapy three times a week for a year and a half straight. At those sessions I was able to vent a lot of feelings and spent a lot of time crying. It was very helpful in some respects, although it made me focus on my feelings of depression even more. My experience with therapy was a lifesaver because it opened my eyes to the fact that there was something more going on besides emotional unhappiness and this triggered a search for other answers.

There were also some pretty bad physical problems that went along with the hypoglycemia. I had fibrocytic disease which became particularly bad each time I had a period, a constant nagging yeast infection, and a recurrent bladder infection that seemed to never quite go away, even though I was taking antibiotics on and off for a long time. In fact, the bladder infection never did go away until I saw a holistically oriented OB-GYN who told me to stop drinking coffee and tea (I was consuming about 10–15 cups of coffee and tea per day), and gave me some general dietary recommendations such as avoiding refined sugar. But perhaps the worst thing was a long-time really annoying case of chronic constipation; it was this that finally drove me to look at my diet, and I got interested in a somewhat natural, high-fiber approach to diet.

I finished college in 1977, and in 1978 really became interested and started reading more about natural and whole foods; at the same time I continued to smoke cigarettes, marijuana and lead a fairly stressful life. Finally in 1981 I saw a naturopath who said I had the symptoms of hypoglycemia, and felt that dietary changes were the first step to recovery. I never actually took a Glucose Tolerance Test, and I'm glad I didn't because I've heard so many horror stories about how much the test itself can really debilitate you. But it was a great feeling to finally find someone who I felt could help me deal with the problem, and who recognized that the hypoglycemia was causing me emotional as well as physical problems. I had been to MDs and they all told me to eat six high protein meals a day and I would be fine. Not only did I not feel fine when I ate that way, I also had to carry a refrigerator full of food everywhere I went!

The naturopath took me off all dairy and wheat, and put me on a program of six small meals per day including grains, vegetables, *tofu* and beans, and other natural foods, plus herbs and herb teas made especially to calm my pancreas, adrenals and all the other organs in my system that were under so much stress. I was also instructed to give myself enemas daily and to stop smoking, drinking alcohol (temporarily) and eating anything refined. Honestly, it must have been sheer faith that pulled me through, because everything got worse before it got better. I had such incredible emotional and physical ups and downs. I knew things would improve and I felt I had to keep going forward as I knew I could not tolerate living the way I had been feeling. I felt bad about 50-60 percent of the time of those first eight months, but the evidence I could see of healing was enough to keep me going. Finally, after eight months of following this program, I began to see dramatic improvements. The next year, in 1982, the naturopath became interested in macrobiotics around the same time I did.

Around that time, I took six months off to go to Japan to visit my parents who were living there. A lot of the food there was relatively processed (contained sugar, MSG, etc.) but I think the *miso* soup and sea vegetables I was eating everyday had a very strengthening effect on my hormonal system in general. I came back in about the same shape physically, perhaps slightly worse, than when I left. But, my attitude had changed, and it was a permanent change. I had definitely climbed out of my pit of hopeless negativity, and I knew I could be happy. When I got back from Japan, I started to really learn macrobiotic cooking and philosophy; and the change was incredible. My moods really stabilized. I remember driving along in my car one day and thinking, out of the blue, how happy I felt just to be alive. A second later I suddenly thought, "What?! who said that, was it me??!!"

Of course there are still things to be worked on. I still have episodes, hints of the old condition to deal with. This September (1983), for example, I moved from a warm to a colder climate (from St. Louis to Boston) and during the winter my cooking became a little too salty, limited and yang. This, coupled with a pretty high-pressured work situation made me a little too tight and wound up. I started to have mild hypoglycemic episodes again, which I could only prevent by eating more often. But when these problems come up, I can stand back and think "Well, I'm out of balance, now let's see what we can do to fix this" instead of getting absorbed back into that envelope of despair and helplessness.

And at the same time, my sense of self-worth, my day-to-day happiness, and my inner peacefulness have grown tremendously. I also feel that my spiritual self has developed so much, a part of me that seemed completely out of reach before, if not non-existent. I recently heard a tape recording of myself talking back in 1979, and I couldn't believe it was the same person as the one writing this story now. I haven't had a bladder or yeast infection in years and the chronic constipation that was a daily annoyance is gone. My periods, which have always been regular only in the sense that they occurred, have stabilized to a monthly event with none of the symptoms I used to have such as cystic breasts, water retention, etc. I don't want to sound melodramatic but I can only say I feel that the "real me" has finally been able to emerge.

Hypoglycemia: Ada Lee

In March, 1977, I had a severe attack of vertigo. My blood pressure (BP) dropped to 70/50 and I lost all motor control (unable to stand or walk). I was treated at the Naval Hospital in Philadelphia with anti-vertigo medicine and started a battery of tests to determine the cause. For some time I had complained of other symptoms (headache, tiredness, dizziness, blurred vision, pains in the chest, and others), but I had chosen not to go to a doctor as these symptoms seemed to come and go.

Now I told the doctor everything and hoped he could explain what was happening. However, every test came back normal. These tests included upper G.I., lower G.I., EKG, ear tests, etc., etc., etc. The test taking went on for six months before I decided to change doctors and went to Hahnemann Hospital in Philadelphia. The doctor there put me through another six months of tests, again with results all normal by conventional standards.

Finally, at my insistence, an Oral Glucose Tolerance Test (OGTT) was done: I had hypoglycemia. I was given the standard diabetic diet from the four food groups and dismissed. I ate only the foods allowed, but continued to have some symptoms (blurred vision and constant, extreme tiredness.) My BP continued to be very low (98/68) most of the time, and I thought this was a contributing factor. My husband Fletcher had high blood pressure and was under a doctor's care at Hahnemann Hospital; so I made an appointment with this doctor to see if it would be possible to raise BP as well as lower it. He put me on a high-protein/low-carbohydrate diet.

At first I responded very well to this diet; little by little, though, I began to have other problems, particularly with neck and shoulder pain. I also noticed a big change in my mood and disposition for the worse. I read everyone's ideas on food and diet, and became more confused than ever! Everyone had a different idea and approach. Then one day a friend recommended a doctor of reflexology to help my neck pain. This doctor knew my problems were nutrition-related, and he gave me Dr. Sattilaro's story from the *Saturday Evening Post* and loaned me Wendy Esko's *Introducing Macrobiotic Cooking*. That was in December, 1980. I signed up for the next available cooking class in my area.

After eating whole grains and vegetables for just a short period of time I was symptom free; and for the first time in many years my energy returned. My life took on a new spirit and direction. Everything I read and heard about macrobiotics made sense. Fletcher's BP dropped to 120/75, lower than it had ever been while taking medication. His doctor was delighted to hear that both he and I had found a nutritional program that worked.

Fletcher and I are very grateful to everyone who teaches macrobiotics. In fact, it has helped us so much that Fletcher quit his job with Hahnemann Hospital to begin studying and teaching macrobiotics. I, too, will quit my job as soon as I can, to further my studies in macrobiotics. Meanwhile, we have begun a macrobiotic educational center in our home, where we provide two to three cooking classes each week and Saturday night dinners from time to time; and we have other short range and long range plans, all centering around helping others learn about macrobiotics. Macrobiotics has been a Godsend to both Fletcher and me, and has given us our health as well as a lifetime adventure in learning about the order of the universe. I am grateful I can share my experience with others; thank you for asking.

Hypoglycemia: Diane Sacolick

Before I became very ill in December of 1982, I had several chronic health problems which I had accepted as a part of my life. The only efforts I made to improve my situation were to see doctors and have prescriptions filled. I was constipated most of the time, usually had a yeast infection, and had between three and six colds a year. I used Metamucil for constipation, tube after tube of Monistat for yeast infections, and antibiotics for colds.

Every year my bladder infections would increase in number and discomfort. After I saw three different doctors and tried eight different drugs, a urologist told me my peri-urethral glands were also infected. His only suggestion was an operation which he said would be extremely painful and probably wouldn't help much. I decided to pass on the operation, and convinced my internist to give me Macrodantin, a medication which had worked for a friend who had similar problems. The Macrodantin stopped the infections and the acute pain, and I took it daily as preventive medicine.

I needed to take Motrin (an anti-inflammatory) every four hours during my period or else, by the time four and a half hours were up, I'd be in tears from the pain in my abdomen. Even with the medication, I was uncomfortable and severely depressed during my period and found it very difficult to get through the day.

I came to Washington, D.C. in August, 1982 to attend Georgetown Law School. My body endured lack of sleep and poor eating habits remarkably well until October. Then I started to have occasional dizzy spells. I'd become depressed without having the faintest idea why. I came down with a cold that wouldn't go away and was bedridden for two one-week periods, sleeping up to 20 hours some days. The dizzy spells began to come more and more frequently, now accompanied by difficulty in breathing, blurred vision, and tears. The only advice doctors or nurses gave me at this time was to "take it easy," and one gave me a prescription for antibiotics. My throat, sinuses, ears, and nose were all infected at one point.

By December, I was unable to read and study for exams, so I deferred them until January. I went home to Manhattan. My family doctor could not find anything wrong with me.

At this point, I was so depressed that I started contemplating suicide. Since there was nothing wrong with me physically, according to the doctor, I thought I must be going crazy. I considered checking into a mental hospital, but I continued searching for an answer.

While I was home my mother had a party and I met a woman there who had been diagnosed as hypoglycemic. She had some of the same problems. This was it! I thought. I took a Glucose Tolerance Test a few days later. My worst symptoms appeared in full force both during and after the test: dizziness, blurred vision, breathing difficulty, crying spells. The doctors concurred in their diagnosis of my condition as hypoglycemia.

In early January I started the diet standardly prescribed for hypoglycemia by physicians—high protein, low carbohydrate. My daily fare consisted of six to eight small meals which included one of the following foods: milk, cheese, nuts, fish, chicken, red meat, or eggs. I drowned my fish, chicken, and eggs in butter because I loved the taste of it, and because a high fat diet was supposed to be good for hypoglycemia according to several books I had read. The rest of my diet consisted of low carbohydrate vegetable such as mushrooms and lettuce. I completely gave up my large intake of cigarettes, coffee, alcohol, diet soda, sugar, flour, and fruit at this time. I notified Georgetown Law School that I would not be returning.

My condition improved somewhat. The depression lifted a bit and dizzy spells came less frequently. Yet, although I was very strict on this diet, I still experienced very severe hypoglycemic symptoms at times. My mind was so clouded that I would constantly forget what I was going to say or where I put something. Many days I would just buy food and prepare my meals; this alone would exhaust me for the whole day. My fingers always had at least two bandaids on them, sometimes three or four, as I burned and cut myself many times while cooking. I became afraid to walk outside by myself, afraid that I would collapse in the street. I stayed home most of the time and "gave it time." I gained ten pounds.

By early March I decided something more had to be done. I began a series of visits to an allergist. At his instruction, I recorded everything I ate and when I ate it for a week; I also noted what my symptoms were and when I experienced them. I wrote down what every object in my apartment was made of, as well as the name of every cosmetic and cleaning item I used. I spent hundreds of dollars on various tests, hundreds more on subsequent appointments.

Over the course of five weeks, I was diagnosed as having other problems besides hypoglycemia, including Candida Albicans (yeast syndrome), an acute allergic state, inhalant and chemical sensitivities, immune deficiency state, an allergy to milk and milk products, and insufficient pancreatic enzymes and hydrochloric acid. I stopped consuming all milk products. I took digestive aids with every meal: hydrochloric acid and Kal-zyme. I bought Nystatin for the yeast problem, and ten bottles of vitamins to boot. I felt much better, but still had very low energy and suffered occasional "attacks" of dizziness accompanied by breathing and vision difficulty.

I was not very comfortable with my new regime, and the next step was expensive allergy testing and rotating foods, which involves eating no one food more than once every four days. I knew this wasn't going to help me and couldn't bear the thought of doing it. When the allergist's assistant suggested that I remove all the plants from my apartment—as mold on them was suspected of causing my symptoms—I knew there had to be a better solution. My diet became more and more restricted and boring as I tried to figure out what was making me sick.

About this time, the Hypoglycemia Association, Inc. of Maryland sent me a bulletin which included a description of the next meeting. Bill and Barbara Taylor were going to speak to H.A.I. about macrobiotics. It appealed to me instantly. I was so sick of red meat and chicken. I read Dr. Sattilaro's book, *Recalled By Life*, and became very excited because I strongly sensed macrobiotics was going to help me.

After hearing the Taylors speak, I was more than ready to begin exploring macrobiotics. I made an appointment with Michael Rossoff, a macrobiotic counselor and acupuncturist in Rockville, Maryland. After the interview and assessment, he suggested a dietary plan for my condition. The recommendations were for food, acupressure points and books—not drugs or vitamins.

After three days of following these recommendations, my six months of dizzy spells and accompanying symptoms disappeared, never to return. I was elated. Within seven months of following the macrobiotic diet, most of my other problems also disappeared. I have no allergic reactions, I no longer suffer from constipation, and this is the longest I have gone in years without a cold, yeast infection, or bladder infection. In September of 1983 I had my first period without cramps in six years. This improvement was accelerated by a series of ten acupuncture treatments I received while maintaining my new way of eating.

I have never before eaten such a varied and fun "diet." Both cooking and eating are a great pleasure for me now. Instead of eating every two to three hours, I enjoy three meals a day. I'm no longer a slave to the clock. If I choose to, I can now wake up in the morning, exercise and wait as much as three hours before eating, instead of staggering from my bed to the kitchen. I've also lost the weight I gained earlier this year.

My thinking is clearer, and I am happier, calmer, and more patient than ever before. At times I do get tense and impatient, and I still occasionally have trouble with fatigue, but—all in all—my health is improving much more quickly than I would have ever thought possible.

Another wonderful aspect of macrobiotics is the cost compared to most alternative approaches to better health. Most of the food is inexpensive, especially when compared to meat and cheese. While I was on the high protein diet I felt so deprived and unhappy that I would often "treat" myself to expensive cheeses and meat. Now there are no tests to take, and no drugs or vitamins to buy.

And, of course, the value of increased energy and happiness experienced through macrobiotics is priceless.

Resources

Further information on the macrobiotic approach to health can be obtained from the **East West Foundation** a non-profit organization established in 1972. The East West Foundation, and its six major affiliates or branch offices in the United States, offers ongoing public classes in macrobiotics and macrobiotic cooking, and provides private dietary and way of life counseling for those interested in individual guidance. There are also *Macrobiotics International* and *East West Centers* in Canada, Mexico, Latin America, Europe, the Middle East, Africa, Asia and Australia. The whole foods and naturally processed items described in this book and in its companion volume (*Diabetes and Hypoglycemia*, the Macrobiotic Food and Cooking Series) are available at thousands of natural foods and health foods stores and at growing numbers of supermarkets. The macrobiotic specialty items are also available by mail order from various distributors and retailers. An annually updated list of qualified and affiliated macrobiotic counselors and instructors is also available from the **Kushi Institute** in Boston and its affiliates in London, Amsterdam and Antwerp; the Kushi Institute is an educational institution founded in 1979 for the purpose of providing more extensive instruction on a full-time or part-time basis for those interested in becoming macrobiotic counselors and instructors.

BOSTON HEADQUARTERS
Macrobiotics International and the **East West Foundation**
17 Station Street
P.O. Box 850
Brookline, Massachusetts, 02147
(617) 738–0045

Baltimore	**California**
604 East Sappa Road	708 North Orange Grove Avenue
Towson, MD 21204	Hollywood, CA 90046
(301) 321–4474	(213) 651–5491
Connecticut	**Illinois**
98 Washington Street	1574 Asbury Avenue
Middletown, CT 06457	Evanston, IL 60201
(203) 344–0090	(312) 328–6632
Philadelphia	**Washington, D.C.**
606 South Ninth Street	Box 40012
Philadelphia, PA 19147	Washington, DC 20016
(215) 922–4567	(301) 897–8352

The Kushi Institute
Box 1100
Brookline, Massachusetts 02147
(617) 731–0564

Bibliography

Abrahamson, E. M., M.D. and A. Pezet, *Body, Mind and Sugar*, New York; Avon Books, 1977.

Aihara, Cornellia, *The Do of Cooking*, Chico, Calif.; George Ohsawa Macrobiotic Foundation, 1972.

Aihara, Herman, *Basic Macrobiotics*, Tokyo; Japan Publications, 1985.

Airola, Paavo, Ph.D., *Hypoglycemia: A Better Approach*, Phoenix, Az.; Health Plus, 1977.

Anderson, James, M.D., *Diabetes: A Practical New Guide to Healthy Living*, New York; Arco Publishing Co., 1981.

Ballantine, Rudolph, M.D., *Diet and Nutrition, A Holistic Approach*, Honesdale, Penn.; The Himalayan Institute, 1978.

Bernstein, Richard, *Diabetes: The Glucograf Method for Normalizing Blood Sugar*, New York; Crown Publishers, 1981.

Bloom, Arnold, M.D., *Diabetes Explained*, Baltimore; University Park Press, 1971, 2nd edition.

Brothers, Milton J., M.D., *Diabetes: The New Approach*, New York; Grosset & Dunlap, 1976.

Brown, Virginia and Susan Stayman, *Macrobiotic Miracle: How a Vermont Family Overcame Cancer*, Tokyo; Japan Publications, 1984.

Dietary Goals for the United States, Washington, D.C.,; Select Committee on Nutrition and Human Needs, U.S. Senate, 1977.

Diet, Nutrition and Cancer, Washington, D.C.: National Academy of Sciences, 1982.

Dufty, William, *Sugar Blues*, New York; Warner, 1975.

Esko, Edward and Wendy, *Macrobiotic Cooking for Everyone*, Tokyo; Japan Publications, 1980.

Esko, Wendy, *Introducing Macrobiotic Cooking*, Tokyo; Japan Publications, 1978.

Handbook of Non-prescriptive Drugs, American Pharmicological Association, 7th Edition, 1982.

Healthy People: The Surgeon General's Report on Health Promotion and Disease Prevention, Washington, D.C.; Government Printing Office, 1979.

Jacobsen, Michael, *The Changing American Diet*, Washington, D.C.; Center for Science in the Public Interest, 1978.

Kohler, Jean and Mary Alice, *Healing Miracles from Macrobiotics*, West Nyack, N. Y.; Parker, 1979.

Kushi, Aveline, *How to Cook with Miso*, Tokyo; Japan Publications, 1978.

——— *Allergies* (MFCS), Tokyo; Japan Publications, 1985.

——— *Diabetes and Hypoglycemia* (MFCS), Tokyo; Japan Publications, 1985.

Kushi, Aveline and Esko, Wendy, *The Changing Seasons Macrobiotic Cookbook*, Wayne, N. J.; Avery Publishing Group, 1984.

140

Kushi, Michio, *Allergies* (MHES), Tokyo; Japan Publications, 1985.
——— *The Book of Do-In: Exercise for Physical and Spiritual Development*, Tokyo; Japan Publications, 1979.
——— *The Book of Macrobiotics*, Tokyo; Japan Publications, 1977.
——— *Cancer and Heart Disease: The Macrobiotic Approach to Degenerative Disorders*, Tokyo; Japan Publications, 1982.
——— *The Era of Humanity*, Brookline, Mass.; East West Journal, 1980.
——— *How to See Your Health: The Book of Oriental Diagnosis*, Tokyo; Japan Publications, 1980.
——— *The Macrobiotic Approach to Cancer*, Wayne, N. J.; Avery Publishing Group, 1982.
——— *Macrobiotic Home Remedies*, Tokyo; Japan Publications, 1985.
——— *Natural Healing Through Macrobiotics*, Tokyo; Japan Publications, 1978.
——— *Your Face Never Lies*, Wayne, N. J.; Avery Publishing Group, 1983.
Kushi, Michio and Kushi, Aveline, *Macrobiotic Pregnancy and Care of the Newborn*, Tokyo; Japan Publications, 1984.
Kushi, Michio and Jack, Alex, *The Cancer Prevention Diet*, New York; St. Martins Press, 1983.
Kushi, Michio and Jack, Alex, *Diet for A Strong Heart*, New York; St. Martins Press, 1984.
Light, Marilyn, *Hypoglycemia: One of Man's Most Widespread and Misdiagnosed Diseases*, Troy, NY.; Hypoglycemia Foundation, 1983.
Mendelsohn, Robert S., M.D., *Confessions of A Medical Heretic*, Chicago, Ill.; Contemporary Books, 1979.
——— *Male Practice*, Chicago, Ill.; Contemporary Books, 1980.
Ohsawa, George, *Cancer and the Philosophy of the Far East*, Oroville, Calif.; George Ohsawa Macrobiotic Foundation, 1971 edition.
——— *You Are All Sanpaku*, edited by William Dufty, New York University Books, 1965.
——— *Zen Macrobiotics*, Los Angeles; Ohsawa Foundation, 1965.
Sattilaro, Anthony, M.D., with Tom Monte, *Recalled By Life: The Story of My Recovery From Cancer*, Boston; Houghton-Mifflin, 1982.
Schauss, Alexander, *Diet, Crime and Delinquency*, Berkeley, Calif.; Parker House, 1980.
Silverstein, Alvin, M.D. and Silverstein, Virginia, *The Sugar Disease: Diabetes*, New York; J. B. Lippincott, 1980.
Tara, William, *Macrobiotics and Human Behavior*, Tokyo; Japan Publications, 1985.
Trowell, H., M.D. and Burkitt, D., M.D., editors, *Western Diseases: Their Emergence and Prevention*, Cambridge, Mass.; Harvard University Press, 1981.
Weller, Charles, M.D. and Brian Richard Boylan, *How to Live With Hypoglycemia*, New York; Doubleday & Co. 1968.
Yamamoto, Shizuko, *Barefoot Shiatsu*, Tokyo; Japan Publications. 1979.

Periodicals

East West Journal, Brookline, Mass.
Nutrition Action, Washington, D.C.
"The People's Doctor" by Robert Mendelsohn, M.D. and Marian Thompson, Evanston, Ill.

Index